Profundity of Bipolar

Text and watercolors by

Philippe BARATIER

ISBN : 978 1 6892 2552 6

To Laura, Natacha and Guillaume,
my children of love

To Deborah, my great love

Don't lose hope,

when the sun goes down,

the stars come out…

Introduction

My name is Philippe BARATIER. That's my true name. I'm bipolar for twenty years. This book to share my adventure, to broadcast my experience. I wrote it toward bipolar people who are entering in the disease and who need advice, to their family and friends who want to know what exactly this illness is, and also to scientists, psychiatrists and psychotherapists, because I give a sense to this illness and I want to exchange about my analysis.

The book is divided in four parts:

- The first one relates my crisis adventures. It's a funny part because my behavior while in crisis is very astonishing and incredible. All what is written there is absolutely true. It can give an idea of what is a bipolar disease, and especially what can be the foolish behavior of a bipolar man in mania crisis.

- The second one is really the guide. It describes the signs of the disease, the mania and the depression phases, and the way I manage the different states of the illness. I also describe the medicine tools I use.

-

- The third one is a proposal of explanation. What is bipolarity? How it wakes up? What is its goal? Is there a way to make sense of it? In fact, should it be an opportunity instead of a disease?

- The fourth one is the conclusion. Considering the overall analysis proposed by the present book, which future I can imagine for my bipolarity? What may I consider? What may I try? What is exactly the challenge?

Part I – The adventures of a bipolar

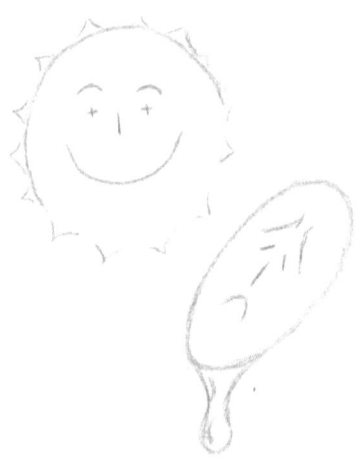

Bipolar, you said?

I am a bipolar man.
Bipolar? What does it mean?
In medical literature, this illness is often
characterized by alternation of overexcitement,
intense but disordered activity, and other phases
called depressive where the person withdraws
into oneself, snowed under with black thoughts.
Often one says to me… "But so, everybody is
bipolar. Everybody alternates between euphoric
phases and sadness phases…" and begins to tell
one's story…

I'd like to begin this book by a very concrete
illustration of these euphoric phases and of the
delirium which can be present at these moments.
One adventure I have lived. Related according to
the strictest reality. You will understand that not
everybody is bipolar.

Travel to Paris

My sleep becomes rare, that is a sign I know very well after decades of bipolar disorder. I call my psychiatrist for a control. She is worried. She adjusts the treatment and advises me to rest.

The day after, early in the morning, I walk in the hills at the "Hostellerie de la Sainte Baume". Few hundreds of meters above, there is the cave where Saint Maria Magdalena would have finished her life. After Christ passion, she would have to run away from Christian persecutions and would have crossed Mediterranean Sea before running aground at "Saintes Maries de la Mer" village. From there, she would have migrated to the East until this famous cave where she would have lived many years before dying. The basilica of Saint Maximin, very close, would keep of the saint's relics. For that, it is the third sacred location of the Christendom.

Floating around the Hostellerie, there is a rare and sacred atmosphere. The big trees seem to be the pillars of a natural cathedral. One walks here like in a chapel. Silence is golden, especially at about 5:00 in the morning when tourists are still asleep. Without any reference to any specific religion, I collect my thoughts, I meditate, I harmonize energies of my body, I empty it of all useless things.

At this moment, I have not any precise idea of my day's program, but I know my state. In this state, no need of any program, only following one's senses, letting the action take place and living it with passion. Until now, meditating phase is closed and villages of the valley are calling me…

Darkness of night is still there when I come back home. Here, I write a letter.

"Dear Prefect,
Communication between citizen and President of Republic doesn't run.
Heavy misconduct.
I ask for immediate dismissal of President of Republic.
Cordially,
Philippe BARATIER"

That was true that communication between citizen and President didn't run and that was true that it was heavy. But that was stupid to ask a prefect to dismiss a President of Republic. The president appoints the prefect, not the contrary. Who appoints the President? It is the French people. So up to people to throw him away, but how?

What is sure, however, is that this action to write the letter and to post it at prefect office makes me feel good. I feel relieved. In a certain way, I feel duty is done. After, I have the idea to go to a television office in order to explain my present political activities and specially to focus on my electoral campaign for next presidential elections.

LCM studios are behind Saint Charles station. I arrive at LCM, but the building is closed. No living soul here. Not so far, a group of artists are teasing about a play they will perform soon. I call to them. I ask them at what time does LCM open.

"Not today, it is the weekend!" answers one of them. "Or much later…" corrects the other. "OK Thanks boys…"

I can't count on LCM. I must find something else. France is in a great danger; I must act without delay…

What to do?

Suddenly the evidence! But yes! Action is taking place in Paris. The devil lives there. It is from there, from his presidential bunker that he can trigger the atomic bomb.

First rays of sunshine delicately lick LCM's façades. I turn around. Here, in front of me, Saint Charles station. And in this station, tens of high-speed trains ready to rush toward Paris. Not a moment to be lost.

I enter the station and look at the departures table. Fantastic! Next travel to Paris in 20 minutes. I go toward the indicated platform. Train is here, sixteen carriages. I walk along each of them until I reach the head of the convoy. First carriage gate is open. First class. Few people are already settled.

I go back on the platform and face to Paris, parallel to the train. I sign with a cross and place a knee on the ground. Genuflection. "Lord, I will need you".

I have nothing on my body except a little red pullover. I have not taken any vest, bag, wallet, or papers. Just a little amount of money in the bottom of my pocket.

Obsessed by my mission, I forgot to buy a ticket. But this trivial detail doesn't come to my mind even for a while. My world is a world of free objects and services, of generosity and sharing. Please don't bother me with money purposes! Minutes flow while sky is taking its wonderful blue color, well known in Provence. A call in the station announces train departure. I take a seat in first-class. A young and nice woman passes beside me. Short skirt and high-heeled shoes. She aims to the subtle chemistry which makes me a male. I don't lose any pixel of the scene. My heartbeat rhythm accelerates. Will she be my prey?

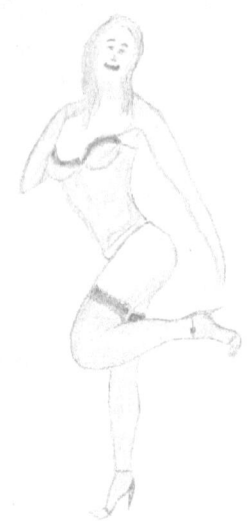

Keep calm! It is not sex time. Let us not forget
the mission. Let us stay concentrated. I breathe
several times with high ranges. Second after
second, the young and nice woman evaporates
from my mind. The high-speed train starts.
"Take care, disastrous President! You will see
who you will deal with…"

At this moment, I don't know exactly how I will
overpower the despicable president, the awful
object of my angriness. But an idea comes
strongly to my mind. I dream of myself
throwing the unworthy president in the Seine,
the river which crosses Paris. Gliding in the air,
and a big splash among fishes and ducks.

For sure, it would be the best way to get rid of this harmful boy who should not stand this ridiculous scenario. I imagine me throwing him in the air above the parapet. I imagine this poor guy struggling in the air before landing in the river in a huge shower of foam.

The train starts, crossing this France I love so much. First Provence with its pine trees and white hills. How many walks have I performed in these magic sites? The best, for me, would be: Huveaune sources, Sainte Baume ridges, Latay mill, coastal ways, … Leaving early in the morning, wearing walking shoes and backpack. Fill one's eyes with colors of May month, one's nostrils with the scent of all these new flowers which proclaim together nature resurrection. Stop at noon under a pine. Take out sandwiches and bottle of wine. Taste the cured ham and the goat's cheese while contemplating horizon and hills. Let the wine do its job… rising drunkenness. Let sleep invade, go away for half an hour to dream land, stroked by sunshine rays which filter across pine needles. Wake up in an unknown world and slowly continue the walk…

That is for lonely walks. Quite a great pleasure.
But walking together, that's better. Especially
when your partner is a lovely young woman
who has a great desire of celebration of nature
revival. Bring one's stone for spring feast. Let us
be rocked by site's beauty, let us be intoxicated
by the scent of all the flowers calling the bees.
Take her hand and estimate if she takes pleasure
or not. Smile when diving your eyes in hers. Tell
her about life of the hills in ancient times. Sing
nice songs to her. Ferrat, Brassens. Find a
location a bit away from the waymarked
footpath for the picnic. Celebrate warmly the
aperitif and generously wash down the salad
you prepared for her. Apples, walnuts, swiss
cheese, cured ham, raisins, tomatoes, rice…

Tell her about the inescapable tradition of nap.
Let her lay down, relax. And there, find the
location of impact, the location in her body
where, with an infinite delicacy, as the plane
which touch the runway, you will drop a kiss.

When you arrive at this point, you can breathe a
little bit. Normally, if you are lucky, she will take
over from you and you will quickly feel her
hands on the nape of your neck, followed by a
rain of kisses, drip first, then more densely like
in a shower, or even like in a phenomenal storm
in case of exceptional spring…

Train joyfully follows its way across France. Countryside of Aix, Valence and Lyon scroll under travelers' eyes. This France is more agricultural. Some cows wring their neck to see us passing. From steeple to steeple, travelers are carried by this prodigious machine which brings them toward Paris at full speed.

Time is counted. In less than two hours, I'll be on the target. I'm conscious of the responsibility which lays on my shoulders. I'm France's savior. I'll free it from this harmful president, from this sword of Damocles which aims on the head of all French citizens. My mission is very important, I'm to succeed.

I know that celestial forces are with me. Even if it seems that I have not a high probability for success, God is with me, that is certain. Else, why should I be so sure of myself? I'm determined, but calm. In depth of me, a great serenity.

Push out the nauseating president from the Palais de l'Elysée, drive him on a well-chosen bridge, throw him into the water. That will not be easy. Additionally, this dwarf, as some call him, is guarded like a precious treasure. Intelligence is to be welcome.

The nice woman with short skirt and high-heeled shoes stands up. She walks in a supple way towards me. Feline, chest pumped up under her blouse, she is cooking me. She glances at me with a little smile. I flutter. It's bubbling. That's testosterone feast.

Be quiet, Philippe! It's not time for that. The woman passes close to me and goes to the toilettes. Be careful! Don't make mistake on the mission… France's fate is at stake. For the second time, wisdom gets over this craziness which lives in my deepest entrails. My animal instincts have been controlled. It's awful to be so sensitive to women's charm.

Now, high-speed train crosses Bourgogne. Around the sliding train, there are famous wines: Vosne-Romanée, Gevrey-Chambertin, Pommard… It makes me dream. France is also that, infinitely sweet things for the palate. I imagine a good meal shared with my best friend, beef rib, few potatoes on the embers and a good salad. Accompanied by one of these nectars of Bourgogne, lovingly conserved and aged.

Suddenly, springing out of the rear door of the carriage, the ticket inspector. A tubby guy, pinky nosed, topped by a regulation cap. He comes in my direction. Not any hope to escape.
- Ticket, please!

- Sorry, sir, I have no ticket. Leaved a bit quickly this morning...
- Do you buy one now?
- Sorry again, I've not much money on me...
- Maybe an identity card?
- Stayed in the car with the wallet...
- I see, said the ticket inspector, one hand on the chin. So, how much money have you in your pocket?

I go through my pockets and calculate.

- All in, it'd be about 50 euros.
- Not much, answer the inspector. You know the cost of a Marseille-Paris in high-speed train?
- Much more than 50 euros, I think...
- As you say, mister. But so, we are not wild animals. I confiscate this amount of money; I send you to the second class and we are all square. Is it OK for you?
- Have I another choice?
- Not really, and don't insist, I'll not always be in such good spirits.

The ticket inspector says goodbye and disappears with my 50 euros. I have not any more money on me. The game becomes more and more difficult.

It remains only few tens of minutes before reaching Paris. I must improve my scenario. How to extract the guy from his fortress? How to drive him to the bridge?

An idea comes to my mind. Knocking at the door of the Elysée and ask for an urgent and imperious meeting with the president himself for a problem related to the security of the State. An extremely serious problem linked to an immediate peril. Assert that the only person I can talk to is the president himself. Wait for the necessary time, but don't give up. Ask for a confidential meeting.

They'll ask for my identity card which I have not. But I'll give them my true contact details. Informatics will easily solve this problem. They will not see anything suspicious in their notes. They'll see that I am an engineer, authorized to work on military systems, with recommendations in territory security domain. My pedigree will increase their confidence level in me and will make my story plausible. Above all, keep calm and determined.

During the meeting with the president, tell him a story where malevolent agents would have infiltrated Elysée and army. My elite corps would have discovered the plot, infiltration should be at a very advanced state, the coup imminent. Assassination of the president himself should be scheduled, even perhaps under execution. Not a moment to be lost. And I'd invite him to follow me exiting by a secret gate for a discrete and efficient evacuation.

The game is certainly delicate. I'll have to convince everyone at every level, but I know I have two allies I can count on, their paranoia and their megalomania. Most of these black birds who turn around the power believe they are the center of the world. They are so often playing dirty tricks on everybody that they are convinced everybody wants to kill them. Finally, the game should be quite easy.

Last meditation in the train. Arrival in sight… Train gates open under Parisian sun. My heart is light, as are my pockets. It's great rejoicing, I hop from one foot to the other, singing. I know my action is beautiful, fair and that I will succeed. I walk along Seyne's quays, contemplating the theater of my future glorious feat and friendly glance at all bridges I cross.

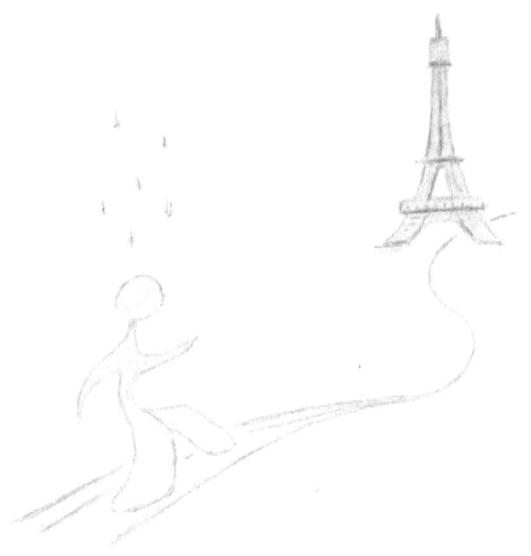

Suddenly, I feel the proximity of a special location which makes sense to me. Here, very close, in the middle of the City island, are Paris Law Courts. A civilization which has law courts, isn't it an advanced and fair society? Here, I'll find some help. I imagine a little country court settled on Notre Dame bridge to summarily judge the Elysée's torturer. There would be many charges against him. Hasn't he ordered the assassination of a famous African head of state for some nauseating reasons? Doesn't he walk against his population will with his unbearable "metropole"? Why does he always set the ones against the others? And my mails? Doesn't he know that the president is obliged to answer to his mails?

I picture myself in the skin of the public prosecutor, harassing the despicable manager of French republic, putting him face to his crimes and showing a vengeful finger toward the Seine. A trial, just a very little trial, not more than a quarter of an hour, we judge him, and we throw him above the parapet.

Perky, I walk on Notre Dame bridge toward Law Courts. In front of the building, two policemen.

- Excuse-me, misters, I'm on a special mission, a mission which would require immediate contribution of justice staff. Who can I go and see?

The two policemen look at each other, a bit embarrassed, then, one of them answers:

- Dear mister, you see, today is Saturday and everything is closed here. Come back on Monday, you'd certainly find what you search...

My head bows. I'd like to share these intense moments with them, people of justice. For sure, they would have helped me, they'd have ideas for the mission. But well, we will not let things get us down...

- Thank you, misters, and happy weekend!

I take again my way to the Elysée. I don't know why, but this idea of plot seems very difficult to accomplish. While walking, I let my mind build other solutions…

Suddenly, the light. Here it is, this time, it is the good one!

Indeed, this time, the scenario is unstoppable. I will surround the despicable guy. How? Using all resources of angriness of Paris. How many are they, these homeless people to whom the president promised the moon and who never saw anything coming? How many are they, sleeping in the streets although he promised a roof for everybody? Me, Philippe BARATIER, I will see all these poor people and I will invite them to besiege the Elysée with me…

But that's not all. Who are these indignant people who demonstrate in the street of our capitals? Wouldn't they be interesting resources? People who want change, who are exasperated by a certain way to perform power. For sure, we'd hit it off with them.

The scenario is well understood. Around Elysée, I'll settle a layer of homeless people, a layer of indignant people, a layer of homeless people, a layer of indignant people, and so on… I'll essentially concentrate strength close to the exits. We'll lock up the damned president in his fortress. Drones, helicopters will fly over the scene and will film this extraordinary demonstration. One will be able to see the despicable president, mobbed by a human flood, obliged to give in. Exhausted by days of siege, he'll finish by giving in. He'll give back the fortress keys. France will be freed…

Plan is at top level. Execution now.
Begin by a precise scouting of location. I cross Tuileries Garden and arrive on Concorde Place. Facing to me, the Champs Elysées open their perspective on the Défense and its new Arch. Elysée is not far, just few tens of meters on the right side. I widely breathe and go toward the republic palace.

Elysée's first railings are there and the president should be just behind. At this precise moment, which woolly job is he still preparing? I'm in a hurry to fight. Though I know the chosen scenario will be long. I'd gather a lot of people and the victory will come because of the duration. It doesn't matter, I'll wait and will prepare every detail meticulously.

Along the railings, there are grass and children playing under their mother's control. Birds are singing and fly searching for food. One of them lands close to me. That makes me laugh. To be at his level, I lay on the tender grass. He looks at me and goes a bit away by little jumps. I follow him, I still go away. Then, he stops and looks at me. Very slowly, I go toward him. The bird waves his little head. What happens? I go to him a bit more, he panics and flies straight on, jumping over Elysée's railings.

Like a ballet dancer accompanying his star, I let myself get sucked up by the bird movement and I arrive in front of the blasted palace. In front of me, a road to be crossed. On the right side, on the tar, a truck seems to be full of electronic systems. Is it for intruder detection? Behind the vehicle, a line of grey cars and their drivers. A black motorcycle, his knight on the back, precedes them. In my heart of hearts, I suppose that this strange cortege is a part of president security operation.

At the right moment that I begin to cross the road, the convoy moves off toward me. Have I enough time to cross? Yes sure, and even if not, why not to show immediately to president henchmen who is the boss here? I begin walking across the street with the slow and confident path of a Lord. After conquest of this little tar space, I decide to assert my authority.

Imperceptibly, I slow my path, just enough to oblige the motorcycle to brake. I'm in the way, the knight toots his horn. At this moment, instinctively, I turn right of 90° and face to the moto. With my right hand, I simulate a gun and in a fictitious way shoot on the knight and his helmet. Then, I proudly free the road.

Arrived on the other side of the road, very close to the palace, a voice calls me. A voice from the islands, one of a black man.

He is in uniform; he is a policeman.
-    Hey, Mister, what are you doing?

I stop and turn back toward him.
-    What am I doing, you say?
-    Yes, it's dangerous to cross like that, you could have caused an accident with the moto…
-    No, don't worry, I know what I do.

The policeman looks at me. I wear a khaki cotton trousers, a shirt and a pullover. Black smart shoes. I have a sportive line. With my short hair, I could look like a soldier on holiday. The policeman adds

- What are you doing here?

I'm surprised by his question. Isn't it allowed to go everywhere in Paris? Am I obliged to answer? And which answer to be given?
I look at him. This policeman doesn't seem to be a bad guy. A good face from West Indies. I wonder. I don't like lying. Suddenly, the light. What? This man is a gift from the sky. There are hundreds, not to say thousands of poor people to be convinced, to be organized, to be managed for besieging the palace. And I'm alone. And this man, educated, smart, able to drive people, able to pilot the fight, falls from the sky for me.

Mass has been said, I'll win him over to my cause and make him one of my best lieutenants. As I'm explaining to him my fantastic projects, I see the face of this man fall. He doesn't understand. He stammers. Suddenly, he takes his mobile phone and asks me to wait for a while. In a coded language, he exchanges messages with his colleagues. Slowly, a cloud of men in uniform converge toward us. All types of uniform, all corps are represented, plain-clothes policemen are here too.

I say to myself: "But what a wonderful little army am I building there?"

I have the feeling that I've been dropped in an ant hill. Everybody talks, notices, exchanges. Mobile phones crackle. Five places little vans arrive and park very close. Stuck to the palace railings, I answer the questions men ask me kindly. I explain like a teacher; I want the message to do its way. Policemen treat me respectably. For sure, we'll become a good team. I'm invited to enter one of the vans. I take my seat. Around me, four policemen. I'm among my family. The vehicle starts and brings us into Paris streets. Around us, outside cafés, along the avenues, I already feel the revolution under progress. I ask:

- Where do we go?
- We'll ask you the questions, Mister, answers one of the state employees.
- Very well, I declared with the tone of a colonel to his aide-de-camp.

I trust these men trained to suppress revolutions. Who better than them could manage mine? Why not trust them?

The convoy stops in front of a little grey building. Two stairs maximum. The state employees go down from the van. Two of them remain beside me, the rest enters the building. A lot of vehicles arrive and park in the courtyard. Everybody quickly enters. A small young black man goes out from the house and comes toward me. Two white earphones hang up from each side of his face which displays a gentle smile.

He speaks to me. Hearing his voice, one immediately understands he is a man who communicates. Maybe an interpreter. He is very sweet; he talks slowly and clearly. It's the kind of man we'd immediately like to be his friend, the kind of man who'd easily charm a woman. He explains to me that there will be a questioning, but that its organization will be a bit special.

Indeed, people who will question me are a great number and many of them belong to secret services. So, it's not possible for me to be directly in contact with them. Forbidden to see their face. During the questioning, I'll be in a little van while my many speakers will be gathered in a wide room inside the building. A radio link managed by the black man will perform the exchanges.

- All right, I said. Go on, when you want…

The black man invites me to enter the little van, then speaks in his microphone.

- Hello the base! Here the flying unit, we are ready...

Questioning starts. For me, it's a big gamble. On one way they take me for a crank, on another way I charm them, and all the gates open in front of me. Because among these men who question me, there essentially are officers. How many among them are upset with the present president? How many would like to change course, to find again France's greatness, its deep desires?

Questions come from all sides. They want to know who I am, where I come from, where I go. I am not to blush because of my origins. My father was born in Ardèche, he is descended from Montgolfier family, flying inventors. Escape from ground attraction, soar so high in the air, that is great. I always have been proud belonging to this genius family. I always wanted to look like them.

My mother is Parisian woman, daughter of an aviator. This man was able to strip down an entire plane, to put down all its components on a white sheet, and to put together again with an entire safety. So, proud of my origins on this side too.

In front of my judges, gathered far away in the building, I truly display who I am. I review my engineer career, my successes, my doubts. I tell them about my three beautiful children, of their desires, of my love for them…

Suddenly, the black man stops me. They don't want to know any more about me, but they'd like to know why I'm here this afternoon. I explain…

The disastrous president becomes the center of the discussion. I say that in my opinion, an African head of state has been assassinated in a suspicious way. What's wrong with this country whose leader distributed so much wealth to his people? What was the real problem, but financing of the electoral campaign of the disastrous president?

I don't see their eyes, their attitude. No feedback about their feelings. I don't know if I must insist or not. I go on as a blind man. I tell them of the manner the president manages his mail, of all these letters I sent him, and which remained without any answer. What a contemptuous guy! Are they sensitive to that?

I tell them about all these homeless people to whom he promised a roof, a shelter and who are always waiting in the coldness. "But, God, we are in the 21th century. That's totally unbearable. Where are the priorities of this damned guy?"
I tell them about all these mayors of France, exasperated by construction of metropoles, of their demonstrations. I tell them of the referendum hold in the country of Aubagne and l'Etoile. The state walks on people, goes against what is voted.

I tell them about my recently launched presidential campaign, I describe my program, I explain difficulties of having to gather the 500 signatures of mayors, which are necessary to be candidate. The mayors are stuck in a partisan logic. More than 80% don't answer when you ask for an audience. Republic is deaf.
After more than one hour of discussion, the black man stops me.

- It's time to conclude, Mister, he says.

I warmly thank all these state employees for having done their job, for having patiently heard me. Have they understood me? I don't know. Yes, I think yes, they understood me. A bit like after a final oral exam, we know if we have been good or not. I feel I have a good file and I've been brilliant. Up to them now. What is their exasperation level with the president? Are they upset? Have I by my speech put the fire in the powders? Soon the fireworks?

I go out of the van and walk a bit in the courtyard. One calls me. A man comes and asks me if I'd accept him to take a photo. Nothing to be hidden on my side. Up to everybody to do his job. This way, for the first time, my photo enters into very secret files, and only God knows which comments accompany it...

A young man and a nice fair-haired woman come toward me.
- Hey Mister! Says the young man.
- What's it?
- We'll move, Mister...
- Where do we go?
- We'll put you in a safe place, Mister...

I look at him fixedly. What does it mean? The young man smiles at me. I think he has reached my side. Am I not the chief of the revolution? Revolution… I search a name for this revolution. "See, let's look at the schedule… The vile president arrives on the bridge, we catch him by the hands and by the feet and we throw him… to the ducks! The ducks' revolution, isn't it a good name for our movement?"

Chief of the ducks' revolution, what a brilliant title! He's right this young policeman, good idea to put me in a safe place. The president's clan will wake up with its damned louts and they'll want to kill me. Why not to trust these men and women who are interested in me and my revolution?

We enter again in the van and perform our way in Paris. In traffic jams, I tease with my adventure companions. Everything seems to be OK. Ducks' revolution is running… We arrive in front of a big building; I am invited to go out. Several police cars followed us. Indeed, my friends of revolution are very generous in their protection. We enter the building, go through a lot of corridors. We finally arrive at a big office.

- We'll have to wait there, Mister, says the young policeman.

I'd nearly have heard…

- We'll have to wait there, my general…

I thank this man as I believe he is a friend of my revolution, a partner of my coup. He lets me alone in the big office and guards the entry with his colleague. A line of policeman look after the corridor. The place is safe.

I relax a bit in this wide room, and I say to myself that the most important part of the job has been done. Message is sent in French society. Fresh and efficient troupes have been mobilized for the struggle to be propagated. Poor people rebellion, elites' rebellion, policemen rebellion. Paris is about to fall.

In the office corner, a bed. I lay down. My soul roams. On a table, a stethoscope. Besides, a computer has been settled on which a screensaver scrolls. Every three seconds, a message slides from the right to the left side of the screen: "Congratulations from Brittany population…"

I can relate to this message. I know a lot of people from French Brittany. I performed my high school studies there, very close from Saint Matthieu headland on a peninsula along Brest bottleneck. Six years among the future engineers, among all these brains chosen for becoming French elite. I have known a lot of these Brittany people, true fighters against our modern civilization, environmentalist among the first ones. How did they succeed, these ancient friends, to make this computer display this message here and now? Are they in the struggle too? Will we build a new world together? Minutes run through the clock, then hours. The two young policemen who guard the door are stoical. Standing up, they wait for a signal coming from the operation theater. I do the same. Patience has always been a strength of mine.

Night begins to fall. Suddenly, we hear a bell ringing, then another one, and a third one, and… That's a festival. Why such a churches' thunder? How many cathedrals participate to this symphonic and mystic spirit? I don't know why, but I enjoy very much this catholic orchestration. But yes, sure. The pope himself reacted! He has been informed of my revolution and he wants to support me. "Thanks to you, Benoit the XVIth!"

No doubt. The movement is in the right way. All these policemen I converted surely continued the struggle. Right now, has the president already jumped in the river? I'd so much appreciated to see that...

I approach the young couple of policemen who look after me, and I take advantage of that to glance into the corridor. Nurses are passing, concentrated on their tasks. I think to the stethoscope. "But that's sure, we are in a hospital. That's the place they have chosen to hide me. Ah! The nice idea! Never will the despicable henchmen think that I am here..."
I lay on the bed one more time and I wait. Suddenly, two men in white enter and ask me to follow them. I don't understand who these guys are and what they want to do with me. But the young policeman says to me that I've not to worry, that these men are on our side. So, I follow. We take an ambulance and go to the other side of Paris. The car stops in a courtyard. It's a psychiatric hospital.

Suddenly, I realize that I've been betrayed. My army is not an army, but policemen doing their job. They succeeded in making me talk in order to fill their files, their famous files, then they confide me to the doctors.

Am I ill really? Who is the ill person in fact?

Certainly, that's not the first time I enter in a psychiatric hospital, certainly I have been diagnosed as a bipolar person more than twelve years ago. But Winston Churchill, wasn't he a bipolar man too? Wasn't he the Europe savior?

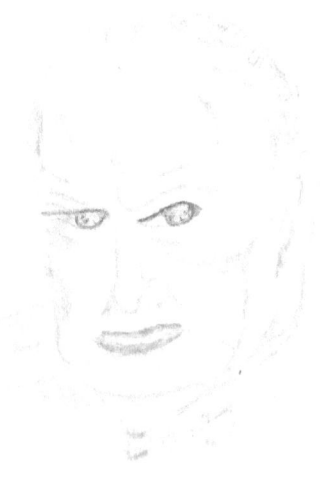

They lock me up in a cell, alone. Hours are passing. I finish by falling asleep.
In the morning, I wake up, freshly minded.

I think about the day before trajectory. Climbing in the Sainte Baume, sacred hill of Provence, going down along the river until Marseille, high speed travel to Paris, but what happened with the nice young woman of the train? Elysée's siege, which didn't last very long, and this strange illusion, illusion to have succeeded... The doctors will diagnose, I already know the result: Bipolar disorder with delirium phases, tendency to megalomania. They will keep me warmly one month or two and they will send me back home.

Back home...

"It's a nice land, my land, the country of Aubagne and the Etoile, a land where the public transport is free. They don't know how to do that, the Parisian people! Parisian people, they want to control everything in our region, but in fact, they don't deserve us."
"So, besides, when do we proclaim Aubagne and the Etoile land independency?"

Suddenly, this new project becomes essential. I prepare myself for becoming the guard of this territory. It means I must think about all organization details. Water tanks. Necessary resources. Speed to be adopted by the group if a danger is coming. I must prepare myself for assuming a great responsibility and I must work on my body for that. Sleep, quietness, just distance with addictions. Lying on my bed, I wait, wondering about all that. Then a new travel is announced…

Third hospital in two days. "Henri Ey" this time. Arriving, I'm welcomed by a very kind man who says he is the mayor of a Paris district. He shows me the service, what we can do, and what we must be careful with. Anyway, silent walking, daily or nightly is fully authorized. With this "mayor", we evidently talk about politics. He says that soon a big wall will be built in Paris to protect honest people from risky persons. He's sorry of that, but nothing seems possible to control them. I'm shocked by this vision.

The "mayor" wants to help me at locating me on the political scene, and to better communicate. So, he places me at the Green center, protection and environment and proposes my emblem as an oak on a white background. More and more, idea of Aubagne independency erases to be replaced by a focus on legislative elections. I already dream I'm a deputy. In these moments, I don't estimate at all the difficulty to be elected on an 80.000 electors district and I'm totally convinced I'll be easily elected in the first round.

An evening, as I'm going to bed, a man calls out to me. The sight lost, he asks me: "Mister, what do you think of… suicide?". I quickly understand this man is exhausted and that his project is to put an end to his life. We discussed a long time that evening and the days after too. He was angry against his wife, against his children, and it seemed that light couldn't come from anywhere. He was in a black hole. I heard him a lot and I helped him at taking the necessary decisions, at least temporarily in order to get new fresh air in his life…

There was also a schizophrenic woman who was hearing voices which harassed her daily and nightly. She often came to see me, to play Ping-Pong, and that was relieving her pain. And this very nice young black woman who was walking with me very long times in the evenings in the hospital corridors. She needed to talk too, to empty her sad thoughts, to restart on consistent basis. I liked very much looking after them. That was good for me too.

Three weeks in Paris, locked up in a hospital. I was walking as much as I could, daily in a little garden, nightly in the corridors. All that to put order in my mind. Walk helped me to meditate, to wonder, to find my inside calm. Then, I've been transferred to Marseille. Eight hundred kilometers crossing France fabulous landscapes. Two nurses for my safety. At stage, we discussed about politics, free public transport... I arrive in Valvert, Aubagne's regional psychiatric hospital. Alice, a tall and nice nurse welcomes me. I know her very well, it's not the first time she receives me. I like this woman very much. She has a great sensitivity and compassion, great intelligence too. She doesn't refuse the relation with a so-called foolish man. They are not all this kind in psychiatric hospitals.

Atmosphere is morose in Valvert. A man died the day before. He died in the canteen, among everybody. The food didn't take the right way toward his stomach. Wrong road. He collapsed. It quickly finished. Everybody is shocked. To be confronted with death is never simple.
In Valvert, I don't agree with psychiatrists. Misunderstanding. They consider my political action as a delirium. Illness. I can understand that my project of locking up the president bothers Paris prefect. It's quite logical that this man tries to put me in a hospital. But the fact he succeeds in that, I feel that totally unfair. Everybody can demonstrate. That's part of human rights.

But the prefect succeeds at locking me up because psychiatrists agree with him. They consider I'm in a megalomaniac and crazy phase. Me, I don't see the reality this way. For me, organization of demonstrations against republic president is a very serious and sensible project. Today, there is a huge number of homeless people and indignant, up to me to organize them around the presidential palace in order to initiate a fighting strength. Which could surely lead to a snowball effect as soon as French people are really exhausted with the power under duty.

So, locked in my hospital, I go on thinking. If going to direct contact with the president is forbidden to me, I propose new kinds of demonstration: Monday picnics in front of the prefectures. I say that to the doctors and nurses, to families who come and visit their parents and friends. I post messages on Facebook. I get in touch with the press. The principle is simple. Everybody comes to his prefecture on Monday at noon with his picnic and tee-shirt. On the tee-shirt, everybody writes what he wants to say to his president.

Very simple and nice all of that, but psychiatrists don't agree. From their point of view, day of my exit looks far away…
I needed two months to understand that I must ditch all these political projects. Ditch or staying locked up forever. That poses questions on the right for the human being to demonstrate, here, in France.

Or maybe there is something I haven't understood…
Finally, I gave in. Forget demonstrations, forget locking up the president. I will be quiet and wise…

And the exit door opened…

Original context

Strange adventure. Not common. Delirium range is impressive, but there is in this story some coherence. From my point of view of an ill man, there is a lot of adversity, but I don't realize that my perception of reality is not totally right, that I make estimation mistakes. And this story is only one among many others. So, do you still believe you are bipolar?

Causes of this illness remain mysterious. Some people talk about genetics, others about reactions to emotional shocks. Difficult to build an opinion. Genetics should prepare a ground favorable to the illness and life accidents should transform the risk in occurrence.

I spent many, many hours telling about my life and feelings to psychiatrists, psychologists and other therapists. This way, I could analyze contexts in which crisis appeared. For the ducks' revolution, there is a political background, frustration accumulated during many years which suddenly focused on the present president. We could analyze it in detail, but it should be better to study the context of my first manic crisis, in February 1999.

I was 39 years old. Until this date, nothing in my life should have been a clue for predicting occurrence of a psychological flaw. I was living a well-ordered existence, an engineer, married to a gynecologist and father of three beautiful children. I lived in a very nice house, entirely built with dry stones, lost in the country of Sainte Anne du Castellet. Everyone was appreciating my calm and sweet personality, my intelligence too. Nothing in the picture should suggest the possibility of a skid. But…

But, the idyllic picture of a quiet family was only an appearance. In fact, in depth of me, there was a terrible feeling of missing, of unappeased desire. I met my wife when I was very young, seventeen years old and we decided very soon to live together. When I talked to my father about my will to settle with Corinne, he answered that this woman was too old for me (she was 21, four years older than me) and that she would be my mother forever. He added that if I committed with her now, I'd never have lived my young man life and that I'd be searching for something forever.

Outright, I invited my father to concentrate his activities on his own affairs, he was divorcing, and I was deeply committed in a sentimental life with Corinne. That has been a very happy period, there was a very nice project of house and the birth of three children which has been a very great pleasure for us. But paradoxically, my father's prophecy went true. Insidiously, my desire for other women took more and more place in my life until the day it became a real obsession.

The psychological pressure became extreme when these sexual urges toward other women clashed with my desire to stay a good husband and father. I didn't know how to reconcile these opposing feelings. For seventeen years, I stayed faithful to Corinne, but I was frustrated not to be able to charm other women, not to hear their song of love. I often followed them in the streets, in the supermarkets, but I always stayed incapable to talk to them. At the right moment of approaching them, my body began shaking, I was unable to say even a word, paralyzed by guilt and fear of unknown.

And then, one day, after these seventeen pathetic years, dam gave way. On the parking lot of a supermarket, I have suddenly been in front of a very nice young woman. She immediately felt in love and decided to put me at her menu. We had a very brief, but torrid relation. She was called Elisabeth. In bed, she was a volcano, fireworks. She was spending all her energy and talent to give me pleasure and that was really very good. One day, Corinne discovered that relation and I had to put an end to that delicious idyll.

During following months, my work took up a lot of my time. I was engineer subcontracting for the naval constructions direction and my client was suffering in a program realization. For a military vessel, he missed an essential component. He didn't find it on the market, and he didn't find any partner to develop it. Every evening, at about 18h30, he came in my office, he sat in front of me, and he told me about his problem. We began thinking together about the techniques which could solve his problem, imagining solutions. I involved all my colleagues in this informal work, and we developed a consistent intellectual activity on the subject.

After few months of this activity, I got the solution. I even got several solutions. I told about it to Bernard, my boss, who had become with years a true friend. The client asked us for realization of a prototype, sharing the cost. That was launched. The prototype has been very successful, then it had to be in competition with other solutions which had been imagined by the big names of French electronic industry. And our little company, employing not more than 20 persons of the region, won the race. A very big amount of money for a very little company. At limit of reasonable domain…

Curiously, the date of this big professional success corresponds exactly to the moment when all broke down. More than this big market, I succeeded at getting another one, very well paid, a six-months job in Norway. My satisfaction was great, my overexcitement too. My sleep began to be rare; I was sleeping only few hours by night. My mind was boiling. There was a rain of ideas, running one after the other in my head at furious speed. I was talking, talking, talking; what we call logorrhea or verbal diarrhea.

It's in this very agitated context that my contract happened in Norway. It was very hard for me to concentrate my attention on the contract, indefinitely disturbed by ideas coming from everywhere. Finally, I produced a very little report which has been qualified as irrelevant. The client refused to pay the entire job. My boss, estimating I was becoming uncontrollable, decided to dismiss me.

The period has been very troubled. A windy day, I felt as if I was a leaf in the wind, I was swirling in the streets of Toulon. Another day, as I was waiting in my office for the final decision of my dismissal, a black veil felt heavy on my eyelids. I talked to my boss about it, and he advised me to visit a doctor. A rest of fifteen days was prescribed to me.

Very strange period during which I was sleeping very bad. During nights, as the little family was sleeping quietly, I needed to put in order everything and I was performing that with an incredible efficiency. When the house had been entirely put in order, I began walking in the night and tracking the boars. During days, I was wandering in towns and villages smoothly searching a soul mate. I met a lot of people, I discussed with everybody.

This way, one day, I met in Sanary streets a nice nurse. I tried to charm her, but the woman quickly realized, just listening to my speech, my brain was not correctly operating. She stayed with me several hours in Sanary streets, she tried to make my wife come, but I refused. She proposed that I go to one of her friends who was a psychiatrist, but I didn't see the utility of it, I felt very well in my skin. She finished by using a trick…

She said to me:

- So, listen, if you want, we stay together tonight…
- With great pleasure, I said.
- I've just a file to drop in the hospital, we'll go to my home after… she added.
- Very kind, Madam! Let's go!

We embarked in her car, a little red Opel Corsa. She parked in the hospital enclosure and entered in the emergency unit. Time went by. I felt it long just to drop a file. Few persons went out of the building and I didn't pay any attention to them. But I would have noted that they were discretely taking place all around the vehicle I was inside.

Then, the nice nurse went out too and sat beside me in the car. She put her hand on the gearshift and mine landed on hers. That has been the signal for the rush. A man dashed into my door, brutally opened it, pulled my arm in order to make me fall on the tar. Straight away, four or five persons jumped on me to immobilize me. They took me and carried me as one carries a coffin.

I was struggling, but this well-trained team was implacable. We entered the emergency unit, the team dropped me on a stretcher, and one obliged me to drink a sleeping mixture.

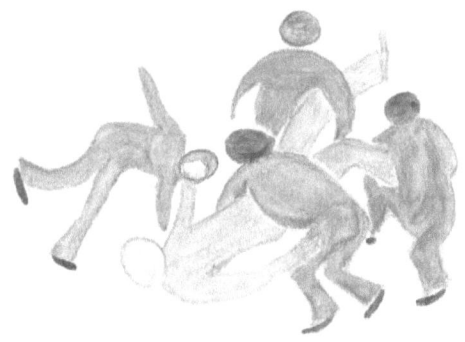

When I woke up the day after, I was lying in a wide white room on a mattress directly settled on the floor. I was totally naked under a white sheet and my clothes were under my feet. I was wondering where I was. I dressed, went out of the room, walked in the corridors. The only way which was not locked up finished in a wide room with tables and seats. I sat and waited a long time.

Suddenly, I heard sound of keys in a lock. A door opened; a chambermaid entered with her cart of magic products. I ask her:
- Where are we, here?
- Here, but in Chalucet!

Chalucet, the psychiatric hospital of Toulon! Welcome to the land of mad people, Philippe!

Chalucet, the psychiatric hospital

This had been my first confinement to a psychiatric hospital. Difficult to enter crazy people's world. Difficult to accept I'm a part of this world I always teased at; I always laugh at. But I must already accept my bedroom neighbor. In my case, he was a young man who confessed to me he knifed his father's belly. There was also this tall gangling man who was always walking with his radio on his shoulder and who indefinitely sought for me to give him a shaver, a soap, trousers or just some money.

There was this other guy who was waking me up in the night to ask for a cigarette. There was also a man whose sight was fixing the infinite. From time to time, he was approaching me and was telling me he discovered a medicine against cancer, aids, cystic fibrosis and even... death! Why not?

There were those who were able to fight until death for a television program. Here, the nurses, well-trained to fighting techniques, came and put down to the ground the fighting guys. There was also this sweet fair-haired face. She was telling me how she had been raped by two men in a car at the very end of a popular town. She was absolutely wanting me to draw her.

There was this big man who came to visit his very young daughter in law in order to give her forbidden caresses. The nurse caught him by the collar, and firmly brought him toward the door while shouting at him: "Don't touch the little girls, Mister, don't touch the little girls!".

There was also the nursing team. And my psychiatrist looked like a soft woman. I was very vivid, and I told her what I felt through my very new mobile phone. These feelings which indicated me directions to be followed. My speech left her perplexed. Much later, I understood that psychiatrists listen to their patients in order to evaluate their excitement level, just for adjusting their treatment.
In fact, she ran the diagnosis. Bipolar disorder or manic-depressive psychosis. It meant that I'd alternate among months between euphoria and sadness, that my way of thinking should be affected, that madness should be invited in my life. Lose contact with reality. In the mania phase, risks could be spending a lot of money, but also, due to an invincibility feeling, to provoke people much stronger than myself. Risks for the married life too because need to charm is very high. Risk to let me guide by a prophetic feeling, as if a divine mission fell from the sky on me.

For one month, I've been kept in this cuckoos' nest. At the beginning, I have been supported by joy of mania phase. I enjoyed these new relationships with the other mad men, I was feeling I was bringing them something. And, with the time, mania excitement chemistry has been seriously impacted by my psychiatrist's medicines. I entered in a sadder, nostalgic phase. I was bored, I impatiently waited for the door to be opened.

It opened. I went back home.
There, everything had changed. Before, I was the brilliant and respected engineer, the one whose advice is called for on every subject. Now, I had become the mental ill, the one everybody tells about in low voice, the one everyone too often asks to take his medicine. Meanwhile, my definitive dismissal had been announced. I was not any more at the center of this boiling hive that was my company, I was not any more the one whose ideas and advices were searched for by everybody, not any more the one who orchestrated the company life. I was like a cargo ship abandoned on a beach, useless and not at his place. Feelings of decline were invited in my life.

That was my first heavy depression. Twenty hours of sleeping a day, and remaining time was invaded by black thoughts. My psychiatrist gave me medicines which just made worse my sadness and dejection level. I had ideas for suicide, I was imagining me climbing ridges road, this magnificent site between Cassis and La Ciotat. A 300 meters high cliff. The last flight would have been great. Yes, but no. I had ideas for suicide, but not enough energy to build a project for that, and to play it.

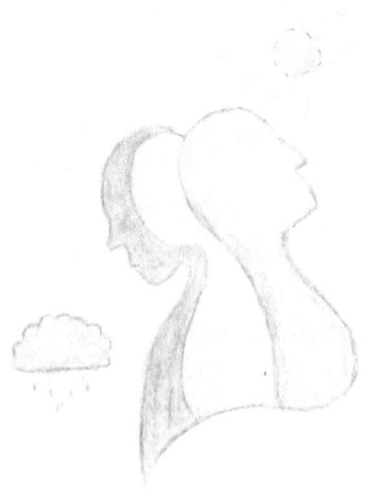

Depression lasted several months until the day I met Eliane. The prayer organized an outside mass and I found a place beside this buxom woman, totally white dressed. I didn't know her at all. She was twenty years older than me, but not stopping at so vile details, she decided to put me at her menu. She was a painter, and on the pretext to show me her paintings, she made me know, in her studio, what feminine enthusiasm means. Explosive and demonic woman!

This unexpected adventure was like my resurrection. This woman's body woke me up. In this period when everybody doesn't pay attention to me, avoids me, when relations with people around me were not frank anymore, Eliane was coming face to face with me and was directly expressing her desire to make love with me. At last, I was useful to something, to someone. She put me again in the life circle. Between my wife and me, this period had been very delicate. Not because of this adventure which had been as torrid as brief, and she never learned anything about it, but because of our differences of point of view about my so-called mental illness. Corinne was a doctor and listening to her colleagues, she was convinced that I was ill and that it was necessary for me to be cured by medicines.

On my side, I was not feeling ill at all, and I felt very unfair and very heavy to have to carry this "mental ill" label. From my point of view, I was not ill, but ill was the universe around me which entered in pathologic resonances. For me, the proof of that was that at the same moment I was confined, one of my very close parents was arrested and put in jail in the background of a very famous political and financial scandal. How, intelligent as he was, could have he arrived at this point?

I was convinced that in our families unhealthy and contradictory energies led at the same moment this very smart man to jail and me to psychiatric hospital. It was totally unnecessary to try to find in my brain chemistry the causes of a familial phenomenon.

Evidently, between us, dialog was becoming infernal. She was always repeating to me to take my medicines and I was taking her recommendations as insults. It was as if she treated me of "mental illness".

I was unemployed, in a great disagreement with my wife. With who could I speak? With women I met in coffee houses or in the streets. Several affairs were born from these stolen moments.

So much that on January 1st 2001, carried by the hot energy of one of these affairs, I announced to Corinne that I was leaving the house to settle few kilometers from there.

A society without money

Let's backup in order to see how an idea emerges from crisis to crisis…
In June 2001, I'm unemployed for two years when suddenly my phone rings. A boss proposes a job for me in Paris. Interim period, interesting and well paid. I accept and move to settle in the foggy capital. That's a period when I'm very alone and the job is extremely difficult. I must build electronic network architecture of a new tank for French army. For that job, I drive a team of 22 engineers and technicians.

Mainly the subcontractors are tiresome. My manager imposed them because of their lightening reputation, they know they are indispensable, and they make me pay very expensively. My brain, after two years of fallow, is very slow. There are many meetings where I struggle, where I have difficulties to follow, where I can't take control. One evening, I said to an old friend: "You know, Jacqueline, this job, it's as if one soaks me in an acid bath…"

But I did my best, I put a lot against adversity and finished by getting results. One year after, on May 2002, for the same price, I succeed at building five tank electronic networks compared to one by my predecessor. My boss is very pleased, he proposes to me a definitive employment. On my side, I better appreciate my colleagues and I begin to be respected.

But I miss my children. I go to Marseille every two weeks to see them, but that's not enough. In fact, that's sure I love Paris, but I'm not a Parisian, definitely. I dream of Provence's hills, of our sun, of the seaside. So, I want to go back home.

At this moment, an opportunity happened. May 2002, that's a very original period in French landscape. The socialist party is eliminated at its first round of presidential election. At the second round, it's easy for the outgoing president, from the moderate right side, to hammer his unusual rival from the extreme right side with about 80% of the votes. I'm fascinated and at a time scandalized. How the left side can be absent from the political debate? How have we come to this point?

The legislative elections are arriving. I say to myself:" I've to go, I've to be on the political ground to understand what happens…" I tell this idea to few persons and I get a move on. I try to build a team.

As a background of this election, the stake is my way back to the south. Aubagne's deputy can share his time between participation to Parliament debate and a background activity close to his electors in his district. The job is better paid than my engineer job, there are fewer professional obligations, fewer responsibilities. Nothing to lose, everything to be won…

Here, what I don't estimate at all at its exact level, is the task difficulty. I think I have a good resume and I estimate that with few speeches and some beautiful posters, I'll be elected at the first round without any difficulty. This feeling of invincibility can be related to my legendary naivety, but also to the beginning of a manic crisis. Besides, in the following weeks, my sleep strongly decreases.

I hardly found a substitute and a treasurer for my campaign. My friends are not very enthusiastic to enter in the adventure. Finally, my little brother Laurent finds among his relations two unaware people who will accompany me.

The inscriptions are closing, I proudly went to Marseille's prefecture in order to submit my candidature to legislative elections in Aubagne. The man in charge of the inscriptions attributes me number 14 as a place on the posters display units. We are 19 candidates on Aubagne, what had never been seen before.

Going out of the prefecture, I meet an astonishing man. He too just submitted his candidature, but on Aix en Provence district. He asked me:

- You submit to be elected?

What a question! For sure, I'll be elected, it is evident... He goes on...

- Me not!
- You not? I declare, astounded. But so, why are you submitting?
- I only want to make an idea known.
- An idea? And what is this idea? I ask.
- The society without money...

Puzzled, I propose to him to have a coffee and he explains to me that barter is much better than trade exchanges. This boy is extremely nice, but I don't see exactly the advantages of a society without money. I felt he invited us to a famous way back to archaic periods. We part friendly, but I'm not sure that, if he became a candidate in my district, I'd vote for him...

These elections are a real battle. My army is my substitute, a beautiful Parisian woman who come one time to Aubagne's market during the campaign. She is slowly walking beside me while shouting:

- Isn't he handsome, my candidate? Isn't he handsome?

I feel I am a sea bream on a fish merchant stall. There is also this wonderful black woman I'd engaged in the center of France. She has a delicious African accent which ignores letter r and she uses it to invite people to vote for me. In the streets, she shouts with her sweet voice: "Vote for candidate Ba'atier ! Vote for candidate Ba'atier". Each time she meets a black man, she converts him for my candidature and put a pack of flyers in his hands.

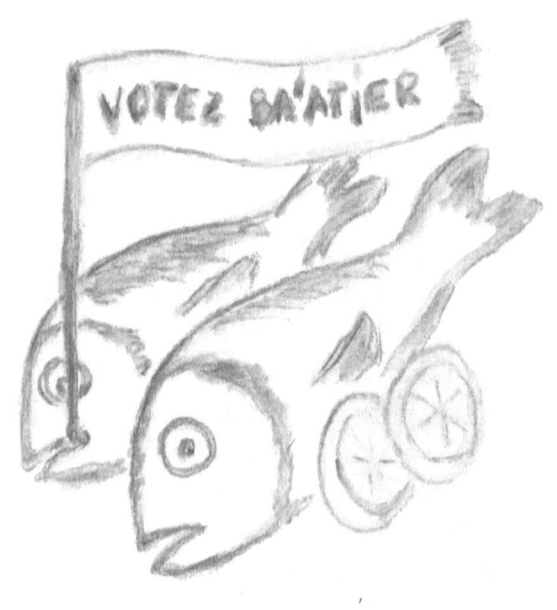

As a free candidate, without political party, I am invited neither by radios, nor by televisions. My posters are covered by the ones of powerful political parties. The only thing remaining is direct contact with electors… but I am working in Paris. Consequently, what should happen happened, I perform the very bad score of 0.41% of votes at first round.

I had spent 7700€ for my campaign. I had spent a lot of time and energy and my boss realized that this manic phase has disrupted my activity in the company. He replaced me. My contract ended. I entered a deep depressive phase.
It's often said that bipolar brain chemistry is responsible of alternance between euphoric and depressive phases. In my case, I think that depressive phases are due to events. During manic phases, I lose contact with reality and I make mistakes which often cause heavy consequences. When I become conscious of damages that I have caused, I become depressive.

After these elections, my political activities turn to sleeping for a while. Later, in 2005, I remember this strange meeting with the candidate who proposed a society without money. Is such a society realistic, feasible in today's uses? Can our habits be turned around without money? We work to win money; we spend money to live. Can we imagine another world?

So, one morning, I wake up and decide to live a day without money. But that means also not having anything on credit with anybody. I want to see where and how problems will come. I want to live it, to feel it. So, I take a shower, dress, have a little breakfast at home in Aubagne, and begin to drive along the way to my job in Aix en Provence. In my head, I imagine that problems will begin when I'd like to have a coffee at the vending machine. How to negotiate with a coffee vending machine? What to say? How to activate its mechanism without paying?

In fact, I suddenly realize that my true immediate problem would be located much earlier. Concentrated on my reflection about the coffee vending machine, I didn't take care to the itinerary and had automatically taken the toll motorway. So, I'll have to negotiate motorway exit without paying the toll fee. An adrenalin thrill runs in my back. In order to have time for reflection, I stop at a resting area and meditate on the situation.

From this meditation the following elements come out. In France, prices must be displayed. But the toll price is not indicated at the motorway entry. Because I should propose this argument, this way of negotiation, I start again the motor and come back to the motorway toward the toll. I knew that I have this argument in the pocket, which makes me feel strong, but I am not sure to use it. In fact, I essentially want to trust in my intuition, to let me feel my way through.

I finally arrive at the toll and a kind woman invites me to give her three euros and ten centimes. I curtly answer:

- I don't pay.
- Pardon, sir?
- I don't pay, I don't pay.
- Hem! Excuse-me, Mister, it's the toll. You are to pay three euros and ten centimes...
- I don't pay, I don't pay, I don't pay, I don't pay, and I don't pay, I insist heavily.
- Ah! The operator says. I'll call my manager...
- As you like, Madam...

After a long telephonic exchange with her manager, the operator invites me to meet her boss directly. She says to me that just after the toll barrier, I had to go right toward the little building. I accept the principle. She opens the barrier and the road is widely opened in front of me. I'd go away like a burglar, but I don't do it. I pass the barrier and go right as the operator said, then I park in front of the manager's building. There, I climb the stairs until arriving in front of a wide glass with a hygiaphone. The glass is opaque. The one-way mirror is forbidding every possibility for the driver to see the representative's face. However, I hear a voice saying:

- Something wrong, Mister?

I don't know what to say, the situation is funny. Then suddenly, inspiration comes to my mind…

- Yes, Mister, there is something wrong…
- Yes? But what is wrong? asks the toll manager.
- What is wrong? Your motorways are too expensive…
- Ah! Mister… says the manager. You're right!
- I'm right?
- Yes, everybody says that motorways are too expensive, says the manager.
- And so?
- So, nobody writes it.

I am taken aback, as the manager is going on:

- And you, would you be ready to write it?
- For sure! I answer.

The toll manager sends me a register of grievances under the hygiaphone and I pay great attention to writing the current page on the toll price subject. When that has been done and well done, I send back the register and ask the question:

- And now, what do we do?
- So now, Mister, you can go.

So, I am free on the other side of the barrier without having paid any money. I just spent a few minutes of my time at the manager's office in order to deliver a message to the motorway company.

The day continued this way. I succeed at not paying for my lunch, nor for my coffee and I am surprised to see that was running without much tension. The society without money, finally, maybe it was not so difficult…

Curious idea this society without money. It entered my life by the mouth of this strange candidate of Aix en Provence and settled in me like a game. I became a true artist of nonpaying the toll and I invented for that thousands of tricks. But, insidiously, this idea was there, in my skull and was slowly maturing. I push the reflection a bit further than what was exposed to me in 2002 campaign. I didn't see any advantage in the barter, too heavy, too complex, and I began to imagine the society of gift. There, no more barter, everybody settles in his excellence domain and offers the fruit of his work to other people. Everybody should spend his time offering and receiving. When we know the pleasure associated to these two activities, living in such a society should be source of great happiness.

A utopia, we can say, but isn't a dream the first step to every transformation?

Few weeks later, deeply shaken by death threats, I enter in an acute manic crisis. Travelling in Paris, I walk on the Boulevard des italiens in an advanced state of excitation. Passing close to a dumpster, I take my credit card from my wallet and then, in a theatrical and solemn gesture, I throw it into the dumpster shouting:

- Good morning, society without money!

Then I go on my way on the boulevard bordered with trees. Suddenly, I want to communicate with these trees. It should be possible, I just must settle in the vegetal rhythm, that means slow my activity as much as possible. I lay down on the pavement and admire the tree's leaves. I don't move anymore; I breathe infinitely slowly. I imagine three worlds: the animal world which I belong to, the vegetal world which is close and whose rhythm is slower, and the mineral world, cold and hard, whose rhythm is nearly stopped. "Today, I'll create a bridge between these worlds…" I was thinking.

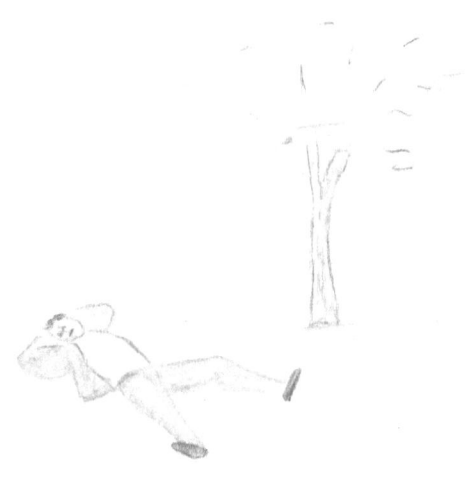

Around me, people have gathered in a crowd. They call to me, they ask questions. But because of my concentration on my activity of worlds' connection, I don't hear them. They worry about me. They call the police forces. They load me without tenderness and take me to the police station. There, they handcuff me, they tie my ankles with leather links attached to a wooden bench, while they prepare the paperwork. Then, they bring me to a psychiatric hospital in which I'll be locked up for one month. All that because I wanted to speak to a tree. Whatever we can say about it, in France, freedom has limits…

So, to you, everybody, an advice… If you love trees, if you love them so much as you feel possible, slowing your own activity, to enter in communication with them, please be prudent! Don't experiment in Paris center on the boulevard des italiens, among all these people who don't understand anything at all! Come in our Sainte Baume, there are magnificent trees, as magnificent as we can communicate with them naturally, in the simplest evidence. And if you want to go further in the communication with them, as I tried to do, choose a quiet place, far away from everything and filled of natural serenity…

In this crazy story, there has been a strong gesture, a theatrical and solemn movement to throw my credit card in the dumpster. It's the sign that, deeply in me, the idea makes its way: the society without money, it's our future, it's for tomorrow. I've just a little time shift, I miss patience.

This idea comes back again a few years later, in 2008, while I want to be candidate at the French republic presidency. Ambitious project, isn't it? Especially when, like me, you have no team, no political party, only an unusual willpower and an unusual persistence. To lighten a bit the context of such a project, I can explain that in this period I wasn't treated by any medicine and my mind was totally free of all these bridles recommended by psychiatrists.

Four years before the presidential election of 2012, it isn't too early for an unusual and lonely candidate like me to begin searching the 500 signatures of mayors necessary to become a true postulant. This quest brings me in August 2008 in the office of Gilles Aicardi, mayor of Cuges Les Pins. This ancient communist is very disappointed of the political landscape in general, and even of the people in charge of his own party. He listens to me attentively. As he is a communist, I talk to him about capitalism damages.

- But, how will you fight against wild capitalism? he asks me.
- I met a man who opened my eyes, I answered. He told me about the society without money...
- The society without money, what's that?
- It's simple. We push the money out of the circuit. And the capitalism collapses...
- Do you want to come back to barter?
- Better... To a society of gift... Everybody settles in his excellence domain and offers the fruit of his work to others...

Cuges mayor falls back in the depth of his armchair and takes the time to breathe widely, then he adds:

- So, you are not a usual candidate!
- Imagine the pleasure we have offering, the pleasure we have receiving... There will be great happiness!

The mayor laughs. He likes the idea. I tell him that before applying this concept in the whole of France, I'd like to test it on a prototype like a little provincial village.

- I understand, the mayor says, where you want to come.

A silence… then he adds…

- I'm not sure that my citizens are mature for your society without money. But, without any doubt, there is something to your idea. We

> will stay in contact. I will introduce you to people...

For his signature, he tells me that it's a bit early and that I must pass again in 2011. He warmly shakes my hand and I feel good waves between us.

One year later...

May 15th 2009. The region of Aubagne and l'Etoile declare free the public transport on all the territory.

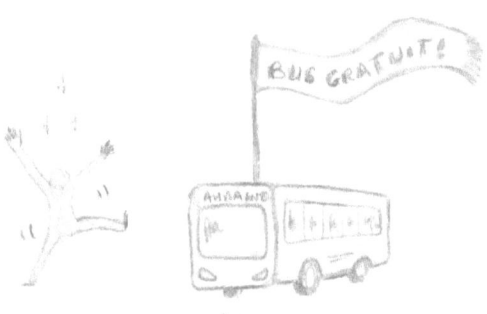

I jump for joy. Free public transport, isn't it a step toward the society without money? I haven't asked them, but they did it, my prototype. Instead of pulling the money out of a village, they pulled it from a whole domain of activity: the public transport. And more, this decision is ecological and social.
Good job guys!

To imagine and to convince

Napoléon was said to be bipolar. His imagination and his ability to convince are legendary. At a very low level, I realized that during crisis, my imagination was very fertile, and my power to convince was huge. As proof, this anecdote happened between Toulon and Aubagne in 2008.

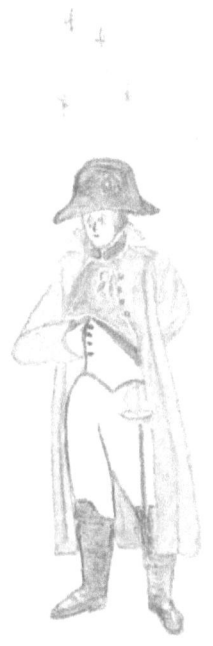

I was arriving at Sanary toll barrier and decided to pass for free. So, I rested a bit in the parking area located just before, time for me to perfect a scenario. It was not the first time I decided to pass the toll freely, and I especially appreciated this art. This time, I'd like to play with the time topic. For me, who was on holiday for illness reason, time hadn't the same value as for the highway company and for its clients who precisely are on the highway because their time is precious. I'd like to play with this subtle difference. My project was to drive my car up to the toll barrier and enter into a never-ending negotiation with the cashier. Necessarily, there would be a moment when the upset toll manager will open the barrier.

But I didn't want this moment with the woman at the till to be unpleasant. So, I prepared in my vehicle everything to sweeten this meeting and to lower the tension at the till and in the car. What was important is that the toll manager, upset by the long queue of vehicles, asks for the barrier to be opened.

So, meticulously, I prepared what could sweeten the atmosphere with the women at the till. I took out my trunk my swimming clothes and a towel. I delicately laid them on the passenger seat. Summer atmosphere. I prepared few sweets and cakes in the glove box. There was even a flask of whisky. Why not?

Finally, I got out of the car and entered in a wide space in which the highway company grew lavender for everybody's happiness. I picked a bouquet which, for sure, would charm the woman at the till if necessary. Fatal weapon, I hid the bouquet between my left leg and car door. Finally, when everything was ready, when I felt the scenario was playable, I started the engine and went toward the toll.

Everything seemed to play perfectly until the last five meters before the barrier. There, suddenly, I realized that the cashier was not a woman, but a man. Unlucky man was I! I was not sure to be able to give a bouquet of flowers to a man, even to calm him. Very quickly, I had to totally rebuild my scenario. And, curiously, I need only very minimal intellectual effort to immediately restart on a new sketch. This one was totally different than the first one, I never thought about it before, and it will be terribly efficient…

Letting my car slide to the toll, I noticed that the young cashier's arm was dangling smoothly through his window. Stopping, I strongly took his hand in mine and shook it while saying a respectful "Good afternoon!". By that, I only wanted the man to wake up and to be open to my project. A bit surprised, the young man recovered and said: "Good afternoon!". Then he declared that the toll price was two euros. I answered to him:

- That's not the problem.
- Ah? He said, astonished, but is there a problem?
- Yes!
- But what is the problem?
- So, a few weeks ago, I appeared at Valence toll and there, "Crack!", the barrier fell on my car and broke my windshield... That traumatized me. Since this tragic event, when I arrive at a toll barrier, I tremble, I sweat, I'm terribly afraid of a potential repetition of the destruction.

Besides, this story was not completely false, because my windshield had effectively been destroyed few weeks ago at Valence toll. But my traumatism was more than exaggerated.

- So, Mister, I went on, I have a question for you. May I?
- You're welcome...
- My question is the following:" Do you control the process?"

- The process?
- Yes, are you sure to know how to open the barrier without dropping it on my car?
- So, Mister, he answered proudly, no problem. Every day, I open the barrier to thousands of cars and I never had any problem.
- I understand, I understand, but could you understand that after the incident I lived, I'd be extremely prudent.
- Yes, I understand… prudence… said the cashier.
- So, listen, I think there is a solution…
- I listen to you, Mister, I listen to you…
- Could you show me how you control the process? For example, we make a dummy test. I'd say you push on the button, the barrier rises, you wait for a moment, you push on the button again and the barrier slowly comes back to its initial position. For me, this should be reassuring.
- Oh! Mister, the young cashier said, happy to see the solution was very simple, no problem…

And he accompanied his words by the very expected gesture… he opened the barrier.
I engaged the first gear and drove straight on full speed, in a huge burst of laughter.
Impossible to stop laughing for several kilometers…

A good program

In 2008, I launch my presidential campaign for 2012. Funny idea for a man who has neither political party, nor financial support, nor team, who has nothing but an exceptional trust in himself. In this period, I don't take any medicine for bipolarity and it's possible that this daring, this excessive ambition is the effect of the well-known invincible feeling related to the disease.

On another hand, the project is not totally incoherent, because the actual stake of this activity is not to become the next republic president, but to use the presidential election as a way to make me known by the French citizens. Then, pushed by the wave of stored notoriety, I could pretend to have chances to win the legislative elections. This way to become deputy was not fully crazy.

Not fully crazy, but the way passes by the collection of the famous 500 signatures of elected people and there, adversity is wide. I contact 130 of them, mayors, senators, deputies and as an answer I only receive everybody's indifference. About 80% of the elected people don't answer to my request for an appointment. They say neither yes, nor no. It seems as though I don't exist. Deplorable lack of courtesy.

I have interesting exchanges with the few mayors who accept to receive me and there we discuss of their problems and of my program. Although I became an ardent defender of the society without money, I didn't integrate it in my project. Minds are not ready; I can't go against the current too much. It would be a political suicide.

However, I introduce it by free public transport. I propose to generalize it to the whole French network, and I develop a convincing case built in concrete. Free public transport, isn't it the first step to society without money?

Applied to transportation, the free approach is shining all around. Ecologically, it encourages the drivers to leave their vehicles at home. Socially, it allows a great underprivileged population to move, to have access to foreign activities. Cost savings, no need of selling tickets, of controlling them, of fraud control. How much lost time found again! What a simple service! What a conviviality! Such happiness is this free transportation!

That is the first pillar of my campaign. I say to myself, that if in my five years of government, I already settle free transportation in France, it would already be a great success. But I go further. I want to set the income of all the political staff, ministers, deputies, senators, mayors… to the mean of French people. Would it not be a good way to make things progress? Deputies wouldn't be there any more to purr while quietly waiting for the end of their mandatory. They'll become motivated people, who are not there for the place comfort, but by a true political motivation.

Finally, the last pillar of my campaign is the nuclear exit. Tchernobyl and Fukushima, that's enough. Let's assume our incompetence, let's stop to play to sorcerer's apprentice and let's take the way of humility. What will we do of all these nuclear wastes? For how many thousands of years will we be damned by future generations?

The great topics of my electoral campaign were so. Maybe there was madness in this incredible ambition. But the project was coherent, the program was correct and realistic. It was even fashioned.

But spring 2010, after six months of unemployment, a depressive wind fell again on me and I abandoned my presidential projects. We can wonder which is the sickest between the political circles and me? I have my idea on this subject. And often, I say to myself that a revolution should be good for our country....

But with age and experience, I don't see any more a movement with spilled blood and barricades. I think about an infinitely sweet and efficient method: the example. What I want for my society, I do it as much as possible at my level. And I began implementing around me a little society without money. So, money doesn't exist anymore between my Chinese therapist and me. I give mathematics lessons to her daughter as much as necessary. She takes care of my health with the necessary means. I don't count what I give, she gives too without counting. This principle runs very well and will be extended to exchanges with my florist soon. Society without money is born...

Passenger of my body

As a watermark of this study, the unconscious. Unavoidable, it is the actual pilot. Sometimes, in current life, we feel that everything happens in a conscious way, that we go on the right side because we decided it, because we examined a situation and we made a choice. However, I'm convinced that a great majority of our acts are unconscious. Digestion is one example of that. Are we conscious of what happens in our stomach when we digest? When we walk, do we know what our feet are doing, our knees, our hips?

In these bipolarity critical phases, predominance of unconsciousness rises at a top level. Between other symptoms of the disease, I have what is called "the mystic syndrome". That means that, unless I don't believe in God, I feel a sort of submission to spiritual forces that often guide me in all my gestures like a marionette. This feeling to belong to a divine order is extremely strong. Decisions fall from the sky, without any demonstration, but with an undeniable authority.

In January 2004, I had a stunning demonstration of what is unconscious, a very unusual phenomenon. Was it supernatural? This story is the following…

Currently, my project was to go living in Saudi Arabia. Arabic world always fascinated me. I had learned Arabic language during my engineer studies, and I was very happy of this project which would make me move from a scholar level to a bilingual level. Else, my contract was very well paid. All that made me very enthusiastic and excited for this travel.

On another hand, Saudi Arabia is not the easiest place to meet people, and even more so, women. And I was a bit anxious thinking to the affective, sensual and sexual isolation in which the contract was proposing to lock me up for an eighteen-month duration. So, I was shared between the desire to go, to discover this mysterious country, to speak their language and the threat of isolation under every shape.

This ambivalence was very destabilizing. So, I found wise to consult a psychotherapist I was knowing for a very long time and who was very competent. Her name was Anne.

I called her to have an appointment, but she didn't answer. Later in the evening, I learnt by a short message that the nice psychotherapist wasn't available for one month because she was moving. No problem! I proposed to myself to write her a letter. I thought that this way I'd empty my bag on a piece of paper and without any doubt I'd see clearer after.

The day after, I went to Toulon and settled in a sunny café of the town center. During two large hours, I wrote my letter draft. Conscientiously, I put down on the paper all the things which were worrying me, which made me feel oppressed. After that, I copied the draft on a definitive sheet, then I folded it, then I put it in an envelope. Finally, I stamped it, then put the envelope in my coat inside pocket, very close to my heart.

I felt as if I was emptied from a load. I felt infinitely better. That was a moment of fulfilment and I took the necessary time to taste it. Then I paid for my drinks and left the café. Arriving to the gate, the post office was on the right side, then a bit further was my car, and I'd have to take it in order to pick up my children at school. What I'd have to do was a wide movement toward the right side beginning by dropping my letter in the post office.

In fact, that didn't happen. Because, consulting my watch, always in front of the café gate, I realized there were three quarters of an hour left before leaving. I choose to use this time at praying in Toulon's cathedral, very close. So, I walked toward the cathedral, on the left side. When arriving in front of the cathedral, there was a funeral procession. Men and Women came to accompany a parent, a friend or a colleague for the last travel. Hearst, undertakers and sad faces. I didn't want to bother theses people. So, I decided to drop my project of praying in the cathedral and to have a meditative walk on the Lafayette avenue.

This avenue is a pedestrian street. In the morning, there is a lot of animation due to Toulon's market. In the afternoon, it's a long and sad street laying toward the port. What follows happened there.

As soon as I entered the avenue, I felt lightening falling on me from the sky. However, the sky was very blue this day. Not any little cloud. A lightning shudder slid from my neck to my heels and at this very precise instant, a force pulled me toward the port. As if someone pulled my shirt in front of me. But there was not anybody in front of me. Strongly. Without brutality but with an extreme authority, this force brought me toward the port. Under the unavoidable control of this strange force, I walked along the avenue for about hundred meters. I felt like I was in a cart and that cart was only my own body moved by this strange attraction. It felt as if I became… my body's passenger.

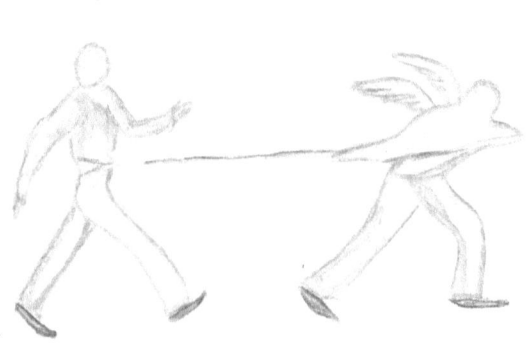

Then, by a bend of the force, I was attracted to the left side, toward a place located in front of a mall. Many people were strolling there. When entering the place, the force immediately stopped to pull me, and my feet froze on the ground. My eyes began to scan the place, to sweep at full speed, as they never did before, searching something unknown by myself. This force which made my eyes moving at high speed was of the same nature as the one which made me go down the Lafayette avenue, outside of me, with a very unavoidable authority.

I scanned the place for a while when suddenly my sight stared at a couple who was going out of the mall. From this moment, nothing was more important to me than these two people who were in my sight and who were slowly approaching me. They were progressing toward me, in peace, one talking to the other. Then, when they arrived close to me, they stopped. The woman facing me, and with a very sweet voice, said to me" Hello Philippe!".

It was her! It was Anne, this woman I had been writing a letter to for two hours.

At this instant, still moved by this unusual meeting, my heart still beating because of these unexpected thrills, I didn't know very well how to manage the situation. I invited the nice Anne and her friend to drink a glass, but they were in a hurry and said quickly goodbye. I stayed there, dumbfounded by what happened. The letter remained in my pocket and I sent it by mail. What happened this day can't only be a piece of luck. Because, even if Anne's meeting can only be a coincidence, this incredible force, this feeling to be crossed by a lightening, can't be a random phenomenon. When I enter Lafayette avenue, something happens, and that something makes me move toward the port, then toward the mall.

What is possible is that, when entering Lafayette avenue, I detected Anne's presence. She was at about 400 meters, in a mall. But by which mean? It's tempting to think about telepathy. And more tempting still when we know how Anne lived the situation from her side. I asked her one year later and she said:" My friend and I were discussing about you when suddenly you appeared in front of us…"

But that's only a hypothesis. What's sure, it's that what is switching this force, it's the fact that inside me emerges conviction, Anne is not far. And in a totally unconscious way. My body knows, but me, I don't know, and I don't understand what happens. Very astonishing to see my body moving because of an information I have not in my conscious mind.

One day, I told this story to a psychiatrist, who said that this kind of behavior could be related to what happens in some car accidents. Reflex behaviors with extreme precision and adequation which only aim at individual survival. Very quick behaviors which are processing totally out of conscious mind, only piloted by very archaic parts of brain.

Finally, I didn't go to this mission in Saudi Arabia. The contract was delayed month after month and I was beginning to be impatient; I signed another contract with a company of Aix en Provence working in telecommunications projects.

Part II – The technical guide

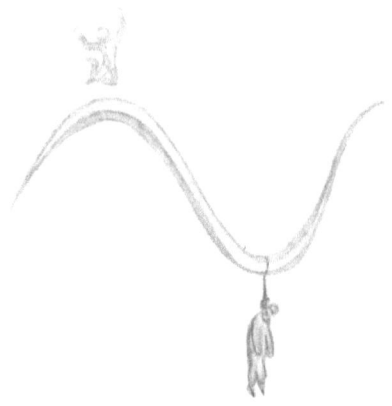

My case only

First, a humble approach. The purpose of this book is not to say that I know everything about this disease. Bipolarity may be lived very differently among bipolar people. Here, I only want to relate my experience, as a specific case of bipolar. The aim is to give advice to people who enter in the disease, advices not coming from the medical staff but more from a great brother who knows a bit the way, because of his experiences.

Manic phases

Bipolar disorder is basically characterized by alternation between manic and depressive phases. Manic phases are very energetic. One or several symptoms among the following may occur and may be signs of crisis:

- Very intense intellectual activity: it means a lot of ideas come to the mind, sometimes simultaneously. So, it's well known that bipolars are very creative. There are famous people: Vincent Van Gogh, Ernest Hemingway, Antoine de Saint Exupéry, among many others. However, I notice there is a difference between having ideas and being creative. In order to create, one must be able to transform an idea into an artistic application or a scientific invention, and that's not given to everybody. Management of the mental state is essential for creation, but I'll come back to this subject later...

- Lack of sleep: Very often, sleeping is difficult in manic phases. My usual amount of sleep is about 8 hours a night, but in manic phases it often decreases down to 4 hours a night, and sometimes much less, about 1 hour a night. This lack of sleep is not good at all for mental health and can lead to mistakes, judgment errors and bad decisions.

- Tidying up: Manic people can't bear untidiness. During my first maniac crisis, I spent all my nights tidying the house in a special way. In fact, my mind wasn't thinking about the task, and my hands were doing the job by themselves with a very great efficiency.

- Extravagant spending: I've not this symptom, but it is well spread among bipolar people. In manic phases they spend a lot of money, sometimes more than they have, often more than they should. And they regret it afterwards. I know a woman who already had a very expensive car. In a manic crisis, she bought two other expensive cars the same day. She hadn't money to do that, but pushed by the mental energy of the phase, she succeeded in convincing the seller to provide the vehicles.

- Prophetic feeling: I have this symptom. In manic phases, I've a direct connection with God. I feel him. I ask him questions, and by signs, he answers to me. I'm guided in everything I do. God is everywhere every time. That's very strange because out of these manic phases, I'm indifferent to religion, I don't believe in God at all.

- Logorrhea. In manic phases, as many ideas flow in mind, there is a need to exchange with others, to communicate. But as intense is the flow of ideas, as huge is the flow of pronounced words. Difficult to stand a bipolar in crisis because he may speak a lot, and not necessarily in a very organized and sensible way.

- Charming and general inhibition decrease. As an extension of the precedent symptom, the communication may take the shape of charming. In my case, I try to charm a lot in manic crisis. As there is a general inhibition decrease, I dare without complex. But in fact, I don't really succeed in this activity because my mind frequently jumps from one subject to another, from one woman to another.

- Invincibility. I've this very dangerous symptom. In my travel to Paris to throw the French president in the river, I've no doubt on my success. The symptom is dangerous because, as you feel invincible, you may challenge people much stronger and nastier than you.

- Delirium. This symptom is widely spread among bipolar people. In manic phase, we often loose contact with reality. We don't appreciate situations as they are. We make

> wrong analysis. We may make bad decisions.
> And we may regret it afterwards.

My son Guillaume added another symptom to the list:

- Difficulties to stand contradiction.

We can see that manic phases can be very risky. But is it easy to avoid, to exit such a phase? Not at all, because our brain produces in these phases a strange chemistry which makes us feel very well. When we are beginners in the disease, we don't want at all to accept the psychiatric medicines which could make us come back in the true world, which looks very sad and boring.

When you are older in the disease, you know the risks, you are more conscious on what is happening, and you often try to come back to reality. But it is not simple at all.

So, the first advice is the following: be aware of the risks of the manic phases. You can have inappropriate behavior. You can make bad decisions you'll regret afterwards. Unless you are a specialist of flying trapeze, please try to avoid the manic phases.

I'll explain later how to do that.

Depressive phases

In depressive phases people are sad, nostalgic, melancholic. They have very little energy. Maybe they think about suicide. And some succeed in this sad task, especially when there is no treatment. A psychiatrist told me that it's not at the lowest point of mood that the risk of suicide is highest, because in this point, generally the energy is so low that the bipolar may have ideas of suicide, but not enough energy to build a project of suicide. The risk increases when the mood tries to rise again. At this moment, energy is present and if the mood suddenly drops, the suicide can become a project.

I have had a lot of great manic phases and only few depressive phases. A very big depression after my first manic phase. I was sleeping 20 hours a day, the rest occupied by black ideas. Feeling that my life was lost, that I would never be able to climb again the slope. Ideas of suicide, I was thinking about a big jump from the cliff of Cassis. 300 meters over the sea. Beautiful end. But no project to really jump over the cliff. Too tiring…

I can't say I'm an expert of depressive phases because I have a very optimistic temperament and so, I naturally avoid these phases. However, I've had a few and I have an opinion on the way to manage them.

I think that we have not to refuse our depressive phases. It's a sign coming from the deep body saying it is tired and needs rest. We must accept this signal as a precious gift.

In these phases, we must rest, wait, meditate as long as the body asks for it. The depression is a bit like winter on nature. Time when our ancient ideas drop like trees leaves, time when we cut the wood, we choose among the branches of the trees which ones will be selected. Some of them will be cut, others will be kept, but shortened. We design the future shapes of the trees, their architecture. Here, we don't do it cutting branches, but making decisions on our ideas, our projects, relations. We drop some in the waste, we dream the future of others.

These phases are essential and have not to be disregarded. They are a part of life as important as others. A well-managed depression can be the source of a new start in life.

Origin of bipolarity

Origin of bipolarity is a wide subject.

Some people think that it's due to chronic brain chemistry imbalance. This approach quickly leads to the conclusion that this chemical disorder can only be cured by chemical treatment. More, this disorder should be related to a specific genetic cause.

I don't like this approach, which is very simple and efficient, but employs treatments whose side effects are not always satisfactory.

I made a detailed analysis of a lot of my crises and realized that each of them occurred in a special stimulating context. The psychological environment of the bipolar must be considered to explain and to treat the disorder. I agree that this approach is time consuming in the beginning, and maybe in certain cases not efficient, as psychology is a very complex art.

But the challenge is not only to stabilize but to cure the disorder, and in the long term to avoid or limit the treatments and their side effects.

Working on the state of mind

So, if we agree on what can be the origin of a bipolar disease, we can imagine that it is very important to work on the state of mind. It means to take care of our environment in order to avoid stimulating contexts. For instance, try to avoid tensions, conflicts, harassments, …

As an example, we may come back on the context of my first manic crisis. As I said in Part I, in this period, I felt torn between the wish to be a good father, good husband, to be faithful and my strong instinctive wishes toward other women. I had arrived at a point where it was not bearable anymore. In my opinion, that is the main cause of my first manic crisis.

In such a case, what to do to avoid entering the disorder?

Not simple, because I was trying to find a solution for a long time. But have I tried in all the directions? Have I knocked at all the doors?

I tried to explain my problem to Corinne, but from her position of my wife, she couldn't hear what I said. She couldn't accept from me who asked her in marriage that now I was attracted by many other women. But she gave me an advice: "Try to have a psychological approach…"

I followed her advice and knocked at the door of a psychanalyst. I told her about my problem with many details and asked for advice. But this woman was from hard Freudian discipline and it was difficult to get a word from her. She only let me talk and from time to time said, "Go on…" or "I listen to you…".

Curiously, after a few sessions, I began to feel desires toward this woman who was much older than me and whose beauty was not comparable to Marylin Monroe. But, always the same thing, I felt desires and it was difficult to engage with her on this subject. One day, however, I stopped talking to her about my life, just to say:

- You know, there is something very hard to say to you…
- Ah! She answered. Go on, I'm here to listen to you…

I looked at her attentively. My eyes lowered to her naked legs which were there just in front of me, then raised up to her face.

-    You know, I went on, I like your legs very
     much...

Surprised, in an instinctive gesture, she hid her legs behind the material of her dress.

Following sessions, she was not anymore dressed in a relaxed way as before. She was looking like a vamp, high heels, black stockings, short skirt. And curiously, that made me dive deeper in the analytic work. I was conscientiously spitting all what was in my heart. From time to time, maybe to encourage me, she put herself in profile and arched her back in a very erotic position.

Did this therapy make me progress? Yes, maybe in taking conscience of myself, in acceptance of who I am. I can say that was the first step. I went on with this analysis for 4 months and then the psychiatric hospitalization occurred.

One day, my first psychiatrist, the one who received me in the hospital, told me that often when people begin psychotherapy, a manic phase can be triggered. I think that has been my case.

How did that happen? Very simple. My state of mind was like a pressure cooker because of all these instinctive pulses toward women. Opening my mouth to the psychanalyst was a bit like opening the cover of the pressure cooker at a moment of maximum pressure. Suddenly, the steam and the food spurted in every direction, that was my first manic crisis.

So, here, one could see an apparent contradiction in my speech because I say: "Try to consult someone before occurrence of a crisis, don't stay alone with your problems." And on the other hand, I say that it's precisely the psychanalytic work that made me enter in my first manic phase.

That's right. But I think in every case I shouldn't stay indefinitely alone with this problem. It could have led to heavier disease, like psychosomatic or cancer, … The way had to pass by a therapist office, who triggered the mania crisis. But, if it was not at this moment, the mania could have been switched on a bit later.

What I want to say here is very important. Don't be afraid, if you enter a manic phase, don't worry. Don't think you enter a disease, but think the bipolar disorder tries to solve a heavy problem you have. I will come back on this approach in next part.

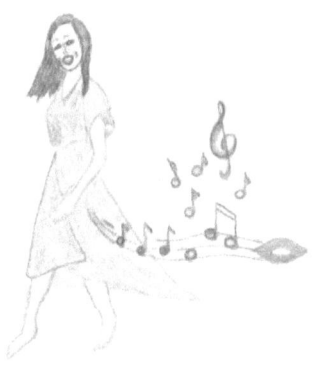

Also, it should be good that at school, instead of teaching complex and useless mathematics, one explains it's not ignominious to consult a psychiatrist or a psychologist, that these professions are useful, even to people in good health and well-minded.

Act as soon as possible, before the pressure cooker explodes, before the cup is full, before the situation becomes dangerous. Here is without any doubt one of the keys of the problem.

Detecting the manic phases

The following chapters may be the most important of the entire book, because they give essential practical tools to live a bipolar disorder in a nearly pleasant way. They are the fruit of twenty years of experience, observation and investigations.

We have seen that the main problem of bipolar disorder is the fact that in manic phases we may have foolish behavior and make inappropriate decisions with heavy consequences. And these heavy consequences could be the cause of heavy depressions. So, it is very important to have a strategy to avoid entering in deep manic phases.

First, we must detect the entry in these phases, and this is not always simple.

What are the signs?

In my own experience, there are three main signs:
- Decrease of sleep
- Intense and disorganized mental activity
- Attitude of people around

The decrease of sleep is easy to detect. In my case, sleep is usually 8 hours a night and when a crisis occurs, it decreases to about 4 hours a night or less. This could be a sign and when it occurs, we must be particularly vigilant. But it doesn't mean 100% a crisis has begun.

The second sign is the best indicator: intense and disorganized activity. Activity can be intense and rich without manic crisis as far as it is structured. It means the mind is peaceful and the ideas are well organized, one coming after the other. As soon as the mind begins to fight with everybody, as soon as the ideas are always jumping from one subject to the other, we must become very prudent.

If one of these two signs is detected, we must have a good observation and listening of people around. What do they think of our state of mind? Do they think we are entering a manic phase? We must ask questions and listen to the answers with humility.

If these signs persist, don't hesitate at consulting your psychiatrist.

Managing the sleep

In manic phases, the problem of enough sleep is critical. Difficult to have a good night sleep; and after many nights of little sleep, bipolar can become very tired. Also, the lack of sleep is not at all good for mental health, perception of reality can become false.

But what to do?

It is difficult to force someone to sleep. If he doesn't want to sleep, it is useless to say to him he must sleep, because he often knows it and he doesn't succeed in sleeping.

Generally, lack of sleep is associated to mental hyperactivity. The danger is there: you don't want to sleep, and your brain suggests to you many activities at a time. My advice is the following. OK you don't sleep because you can't, but don't let your brain bring in a lot of various activities at a time. Have a rest, try to rest as much as possible, relax. Lay on your bed if you can. Sometimes, take a shower or a bath. Listen to sweet music. Keep calm. Breathe well.

You can also ask a psychiatrist for specialized medicine. In my case, Theralene is often prescribed by my psychiatrist, but it is not always effective.

Managing the serenity

More than the amount of sleep, mind serenity is essential.

How to pass from a state where a lot of ideas cross the brain in every sense to another one, wise and peaceful?

The main tool for that is for sure the meditation. This activity is well known by societies for centuries. There could be different schools of thought, but the aim is always the same: find again peace of mind.

How does it work?

Very simple. Find a calm and relaxing place and breathe widely several times before beginning. Then let the ideas come in your mind, welcome them, accept them but don't process them. For each idea coming to your mind, just say hello to it and very quickly goodbye to it. Don't enter in a deep reflection on the idea.

I practice this technique several times a day in a garden near my house and that's very efficient to feel relaxed and peaceful.

Another topic is the management of the environment. Try to not be bothered every time by toxic people who submerge you under their problems without respecting you. Choose the right persons to be your friends and manage the relations with your family in order to get the best for and from them.

Sport could also be very good. I walk a lot and that is essential for my serenity.

Another very important thing is the place where you live. Bipolar needs calm. I can say that in manic crisis, it's better to be alone. Because your nights are shorter, and to compensate, you may need to have a nap at every moment of the day. The best is to accept the sleep when it comes. Because also, you need not to be disturbed by non-appropriate chatter. You are in a phase where you need to think about yourself and you have not to solve problems of everybody. So, in manic phases, it's better to live alone, or to live with a very smart and respectful person.

Invalidity or not?

In France, a psychiatrist can ask the government for an invalidity pension for a bipolar. In certain cases, it can be accepted. I have such a pension for about ten years. Before that, I tried to live my bipolar disorder while working in software engineering companies as a project manager.

But that was very difficult. In ten tears, I moved ten times and I had three job dismissals. Finally, it was not efficient at all. Each time, I was entering a company and learning their specific activity for months or years, and just when I began to be efficient at the job, I entered in a manic phase and was systematically dismissed.

Difficult to manage a crisis while performing a job with responsibility. Finally, I asked for a pension and I got it. I have no shame for that. Without any doubt, I'm more useful to society in this way of life than the one before. Do you want proof? You have it under your eyes. I've time to write a book, to share my experience…

When I stopped working, without any doubt, that improved my health status. Fact not to be exposed to industrial environment stress, schedules pressure, angriness of others, offered a life of quality, favorable to my stabilization. For sure, this leaves a great void, but I filled it by various activities paid or not: cooking for homeless people, creation of a footpath, bipolar association management, mathematics teaching and writing, …

So, if you remember my advices on the management of sleep and serenity, it's nearly impossible to do it while working. In my opinion, if you have a severe bipolar disorder, don't hesitate to ask for an invalidity pension and enjoy your new way of life.

Albert Einstein's method

As we talk about mind management and meditation, I'll tell you an interesting story about Albert Einstein's way of life. I read one of his books long ago, and in its first chapter, the scientist was describing his work method.

In fact, he said he was working with the same method as Sherlock Holmes, the famous detective. And how did he work, Sherlock Holmes?

Very simple. He began his investigation by going out, collecting clues, interrogating people and analyzing documents. Albert Einstein says that in this phase the detective works a lot, it is the compression phase.

After that, he went back home, sat in an armchair, fired a pipe and relaxed. He doesn't try to solve the problem anymore, but only lets his mind relax. This is what he calls the decompression phase. And what happens?

Very often, in the decompression phase, ideas and pieces of solution suddenly appear. No effort from the mind to get the solutions which automatically emerges from the brain.

Sherlock Holmes enjoys the fact he found a part of the solution and enters into a new compression phase to go further. Then, a new decompression phase. So, by an iteration process, the detective approaches the solution more and more.

Albert Einstein used this method and often played violin in decompression phases. Everyone knows the success of his works.

I employ this method too and I enjoy it a lot. I alternate between compression and decompression phases according to my own body rhythm. Generally, about two hours of work, and one hour of meditation in the garden. I stop the work phases when I begin to be intellectually tired or when I make little and frequent mistakes. Working according to one's own rhythm is the source of great pleasure.

So, it is important to understand the power of relaxation. It is not necessary to persist in working all the time to get results. Alternating activity phases with relaxation phases could be much more efficient and for sure more pleasant.

A tool: the medicines

I have been fighting against medication for a long time. As I didn't feel ill, I thought it was not necessary for me to take any medicine. In my opinion, the ill component was not me, but the overall society around me, which I found very pathologic. The society had to be cured, not me.

As I explained before, the subject of medicines was very critical and may have been the main reason of my divorce with Corinne. This subject was very destabilizing for me. Why? Because when I didn't take medicines, everyone around me, family and close friends worried about me. And they believed that was good for me and many of them were telling me about medicines all day long. They were saying: "Be careful, Philippe, you are on a foolish slope, you are losing control, you must take your medicines."

In fact, their speech telling me I was becoming foolish, coming from every side, made me crazy. It was very difficult to stand, and my reaction was to go away just to find a place where people should be gentle with me. Or a desert place.

One day, I understood a very important thing. If you take your medicine, you calm family and friends. And instead of a permanent harassment, all of them become very quiet and friendly with you. This boomerang effect brings you back quietness and calm, it becomes easier to manage the crisis. A bit later, I began to feel effects of the medicine on my health, on crisis control, which became less and less frequent, or could totally vanish. What a comfort! How could I not enjoy this luxury for so many years?

But despite these undisputable benefits, I'm not really convinced by medicines. I take it as a tool, not as a religion. It's a bit like dressing on a cut. It's not done to last forever. First because of side effects on the liver, the kidney, libido and inspiration. Then because the man must not live bridled. I'd like to recover my ancient sexuality, the one I meet sometimes in crisis, enhanced, volcanic, magnificent…

My treatment

Since my first confinement in 1999, I've tried a lot of medicines:

- Solian,
- Depakote,
- Depamide,
- Tégrétol,
- Abilify,
- Lithium,
- Risperdal

Plus, special treatment for manic crisis control. From 1999 to 2011, I was not really convinced by benefits of treatment, so, I didn't take a great care of medicine. Sometimes, I took them and sometimes not. That is not efficient at all. In the beginning when crisis will occur, I decided to stop the treatment. That could explain why the results were not perfect…

In 2011, after a great crisis in which I tried to throw the president of republic in the Seine, I said:" Now, that's enough! I have to take my problem in my own hands." I decided to stop moving and bought a little apartment in Aubagne. I decided also to find a good treatment for my health.

My psychiatrist and I needed two years to find the right components and the right dosages of the medicines. Since 2013, we can say we have found a good balance. So, the treatment is now:
- Lithium. The lithium is a mood regulator, it avoids having high and low spirits.
- Risperdal, a neuroleptic which role is to avoid being delirious.

Moreover, when a crisis occurs, to recover calm and quietness, I use Locsapac, which is very efficient, but has very uncomfortable zombie like side effects, and also Theralene, which helps sleeping.

Anyway, I'm stabilized for six years. Not any more confinements, not any more spectacular delirium, the wild animal is under control! That doesn't mean vigilance flags. Now, I know the symptoms of crisis: a significant decrease of sleep, feverish states of mind, mental activity jumping from one subject to another, intellectually bubbling with excitement. As soon as one of these signs appears, I consult my psychiatrist and we adjust the treatment. I postpone all the tasks which are not indispensable and, even if I don't succeed in sleeping, I dive into a state of deep relaxation.

That is possible because of my invalid status. So, all that means is that the psychiatric team and I have made good progress in crisis management. These medicines are not without side effects. Lithium may cause damage on kidney function, which must be monitored. And the Risperdal? My psychiatrist confessed to me one day that it is a testosterone inhibitor, the male hormone. That means that my libido is weakened. Sexual life becomes more complicated, less spontaneous, less burning. Inspiration too suffers from this medicine which, fighting against delirium, also fights against imaginative function as a side effect.

Risperdal dosage is always a subject of delicate negotiation between my psychiatrist and I. Often, when my sexual performances decrease or when my inspiration is very bad, I ask her to decrease this medicine dosage. She generally accepts, but always recalling that as soon as the first little sign of crisis occurs, we increase the dosage back. Most of the time, treatment decrease is effective. I become more sensitive to feminine charm, I more often want them, and the sexual mechanics has more according with what is required by the function… My inspiration is better for writing, but with a great freedom. That means it's not always easy to focus on a given subject or on the purpose of the book I'm writing.

Few weeks after, generally less than two months, first signs of crisis appear. My mind, unless agile, becomes crowded by many very magnificent ideas and projects. These beginnings of crisis are very prolific periods which very often lead to original concepts. These concepts will be useful later when peace and calm will have been reconquered. Sleep becomes rare, I've to consult my psychiatrist, to increase the treatment.

I'll explain in Part IV which are my projects about treatment.

A tool: the psychiatric hospital

The psychiatric hospital has a bad reputation. That is not fair. Hospital is a quiet place where you can rest, protected by the medical staff. Generally, there is a garden you can walk in. You can also have activities if you want.

If you need, you can discuss with nurses, and if you are patient, with psychiatrists.

An advantage of the hospital is that it takes you away from your usual context. And, in many cases, crisis may have its cause in your relation to this context (family and work, …). Far away from the source of your problems, you can take time to meditate, to find solutions and to make decisions about your problem.

In the hospital, we meet a lot of people and we have time to talk to them, to listen to them. I've made many friends in the hospital. I've had a great love story too, a very beautiful relation which lasted seven years.

Finally, it's a place where a lot of pathology are concentrated and it's very instructive to learn about it. It can help at understanding our own behavior.

So, if necessary, don't hesitate to ask your psychiatrist for a place in the hospital.

How to live a crisis?

Crises are often euphoric. We feel beautiful, intelligent, invincible. Contacts are many, easy and rich. We think everything is possible. God is our friend, he is everywhere, he is guiding us, and this feeling is very pleasant. Projects come from everywhere, there are many ideas, it's a bit like if we were at the cinema. How not to enjoy such a context?

One says to you:" You're ill!" and you don't understand, the world has never been so nice for you. You are not ill; you are probably curing of something. Anyway, your unconscious tries new ways to solve a problem. I'll explain in Part III with many details what I mean.

Don't refuse your crisis, don't refuse its symptoms. Accept it, it's the way your body chooses to talk. But don't overeat your crisis, refuse the demoniac rhythm your body would impose, breathe, rest, live your crisis slowly, taste it, feed yourself of what it wants to bring you. Appreciate it as the most delicious of the nectars.

Look after your sleep, and if you don't succeed in sleeping, take time to rest, to relax, to meditate. Listen to sweet music, take baths or showers, have littles walks in the country. Isolate if you see there are conflicts with people around you. Pay a great attention to this important period of your life. Live it entirely! Taste it!

Don't stay alone in front of your problems!

Bipolar friends, if I only give one advice to you, it would be: "Talk!". Don't stay alone in front of problems which are mining you. Don't let yourself invade, submerge, or become dominate by frustrations which keep coming. And the advice is also valid for those which bipolar disorder didn't already touch. Unsolved psychological problems which indefinitely come on the table are fertile ground for mental illness.

If you can talk to a friend, someone close to you, of what is heavy in your heart, of what tarnishes your life, you're lucky. This happiness is not given to everybody. In this second case, try to consult a psychiatrist, a psychologist, or a therapist as there are many now. Find the person who is the best for you and do the job you need. Talking, you'll understand what happens to you, and you'll live it better. It's the first step toward therapy…

For some people, therapy cost is a heavy problem. But it's well known that, in France, consultations with psychiatrists are widely refunded by social security and health mutual. In medical psychological centers (CMP), sessions with psychologists and psychotherapists are totally free. Sometimes, there are also free sophrology sessions, which are very good for mental health.

Then, there are bipolar who don't want at all to be in contact with doctors or medical environment. For these people, there are mutual help groups (Groupes d'entraide mutuelle / GEM). These independent associations offer various activities to people touched by mental illness (depressive, bipolar, schizophrenic, …). That creates social link. No caregiver is accepted in these structures. Ill people exchange between themselves about their life and disease.

I was proud to create and be president of such a GEM in Aubagne in 2011. It was called "La Montgolfière". Every week, we brought ill people in the hills, to breathe a bit while walking or sharing a picnic. This had been a very rich experience. During summer, we went to free shows and concerts in the region and everybody was happy.

A word toward family and friends

You, families of bipolar, friends, colleagues, you are the true victims of bipolarity!

In the beginning, you don't know what happens, you see your husband, your brother, your father behaving very differently than usual. You worry, mainly for him. You are afraid that he acts inappropriately, that he spends his money without any count, that dishonest people cheat him, that he takes high risks and puts his life in danger. You don't arrive to talk to him anymore, to listen to him. Misunderstanding is the rule.

You consult a psychiatrist and the verdict falls. Hospitalization is necessary. But there is a problem, he doesn't want at all to be confined, freedom is so beautiful. So, you must trigger the hospitalization procedure. The hunt begins. As a dangerous tawny, he is tracked, circled. Finally, he is caught, tied to be driven to the hospital.

My wife, Corinne did that, and my two daughters, Laura and Natacha, just out of the teen age, had also to pilot this subtle operation. One after the other. Because they love me. When it occurred, I was very upset, but with hindsight, I'm infinitely grateful to them. These three women are exceptional persons, they protected me against my will. It was the voice of intelligence and wisdom.

I think the family has an important role to play in bipolarity, essentially in crises prevention. It's more difficult to repair the dam when it gives in. All of us are potentially bipolar and we live in the world of competition and isolation. Everybody must solve his own problems and that is the most critical point. Let us learn mutual help, let us really listen to what the other says and let us know how to detect people who are submerged by unbearable interior conflicts. Let us help them to manage their difficulty to live, let us share our life experiences. And if that is not enough, if the problem is really critical, apparently without solution, let us not hesitate at consulting professionals.

Part III – Bipolarity: an opportunity?

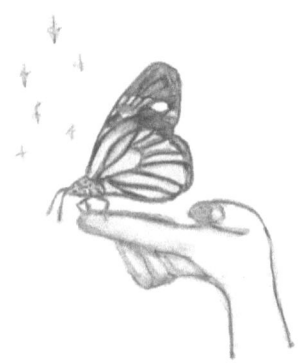

Contexts of crises occurrence

Bipolar crisis often destroys familial and professional lives. So, crisis is often considered as negative item. But experience showed me that crisis may often be a very efficient tool.

I said in Part II (chapter Origin of bipolarity) that in my opinion, bipolar disorder is not only due to a chronic brain chemistry imbalance, but that it can be associated to contexts. I made a detailed analysis of several of my crises and concluded that in each of them, I had to face difficult problems apparently without solutions.

My proposal is:

"Bipolarity is only a way to open resolution of unsolved problems to new approaches."

So, we'll debrief hereafter three of my crises in order to identify in each case what was the problem and how bipolarity found a solution to it. The three selected crises are:
-    The first one,
-    The most spectacular one,
-    The last one.

Debriefing on a charming husband

I described in detail in Part I (Original context) my first manic crisis and its context. In this period, I was trapped between two antagonistic wishes. On one side, I wanted to charm all the women on the earth and make love with them. On the other hand, I wanted to stay a good father, and a faithful good husband. I was totally unable to gather these two parts of me.

This internal conflict created tensions and led to inappropriate behavior. For instance, when I was with my wife, I very often thought about other women. But when I tried to charm other women, following them in the streets, I was totally unable to speak to them, paralyzed by guilt.

For many years, I was torn between these incompatible wishes. I tried a lot of things, without any success. What happened?

One day, my body said" Stop! We'll not indefinitely stay in this unsuccessful attitude. Let us allow a new way of behavior…" and it allowed me, among a multitude of other permissions, to discuss with women in the streets. It totally disinhibited me on the subject as far as the nurse I met in Sanary. She had the surprise to see me singing songs for her while lying on the pavement.

The new way allowed by bipolarity was typically in the madness field. That's the principle of bipolarity action. Opening the investigation field to madness.

What happened?

I've been brought to a psychiatric hospital. There, I met psychotherapists and put under the lights this problem which was eating me for seventeen years. Crisis made my problem pass from a secret and unspoken domain to a public one which everyone can tell about. It trivialized it; it unloaded the relative affective load. Crisis pushed me to unemployment, which gave me time to meditate on the question, and time to meet other women and maybe to progress on the problem. Finally, crisis led me to meet several therapists and one of them one day advised me to leave the family house in order to build a personal space. That has been a true beginning…

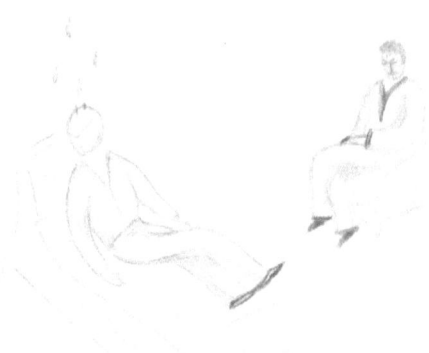

So, I say that the crisis allowed to escape from the pathetic purr I felt inside, to enter a new life, which would not be easier, but which, in every case, proposed some opportunities.

Debriefing on a failed coup

I began this book by telling you the story of a failed coup. When I tell this story to people, there are two types of reaction. Some say:" But guy, you aren't foolish at all. It should be the contrary. What a heroic and savior act for humanity! Listen, next time you do that, call me, I'll come with you…" Others, embarrassed, turn their tongue seven times in their mouth before dropping few words of admiration toward the president who had been my target, not understanding how I could hate him so much. I want to talk to these people. Maybe this hate could look pathologic, but I'll explain on which ground it is built.

Everything begins during an evening of presidential election with my first daughter Laura. We have voted left, the right-side wins. Laura's heart always beats on the left side and she is militant for the true causes. Here, she is dismayed. She asks me what I think about the situation. I say:

- We have lost. It's the democratic game. We now have a new president; I'll Love him because French people elected him…
- How can you say such crazy things, Dad? You know who he is, this one? She answers.

It's this way, I welcome the president. It was cordial but not warm…

One year passed. I was evolving along my Russian mountains, and my present psychiatrist tried to cure me with Tégrétol. I loved this little man very much. He always had relevant remarks, an acute intelligence, and a lot of interesting stories to be told…

In this period, I met for the first time a Chinese medicine practitioner. She practiced acupuncture on me and prescribed Chinese medicine which would normally cure me from bipolarity. The cost of this therapy was:
-    Two acupuncture sessions (2 x 45 €)
-    Chinese medicine (50 €)

So, that meant that with about 140€, you can say bye bye to bipolarity.

It was impressive! I had followed the indications for one month and the practitioner declared to me using a confident tone: "Philippe, you are cured!". I found that fabulous. I felt cured, but was I really cured?

I found that so wonderful that I told a friend about it. He was in a very high position in French medical power. I asked him if authorities would finance studies on efficiency of Chinese medicine on bipolar disorder. Because, if on one hand the success was real, the social security would save a lot of money in medicines, consultations and hospitalizations. But on the other hand, if the Chinese therapy was an illusion, it would be useful to punish the faults.

He listened to me attentively, then he said to me:" Don't waste your time! All the decision makers of the health chain are feasting on psychiatry. They will not cut the branch on which they seat. Chinese medicine will do its way at its rhythm. Let it take necessary time to convince…"

I was scandalized, essentially because I knew the professional position of my friend, and I wondered who could have a more acute and more relevant view on the situation. What to do if the overall health chain was corrupted? Who can go against that? Who can impose a scientific and pragmatic approach of the medicine?

Who?

Yes! For sure, the president of the republic.

So, I wrote to the president a letter asking for a scientific study about efficiency of Chinese medicine against bipolarity. His chief of staff immediately answered me that he was transferring the file to the Ministry of Health and that I'll be informed.

I waited. I waited one year and half, until February 2010. Ministry of Health didn't send any sign of life and, as the president didn't give me any name as a contact in this administration, it was up to him to endure the fruit of my impatience.

So, I send him a second letter, more original. I carefully packed my pipe and I mailed it. I refreshed president's memory about our precedent exchange. I told him that apparently it was difficult to be understood, but that he only had to put this pipe somewhere, to propose a date, an hour, and that I'd meet him with pleasure.

This time, he didn't answer. But, a few weeks after, a strange coincidence happened.

At this time, I worked at Eurocopter, European leader for helicopter design and production. I was an expert in simulation of some essential functions of the NH90. Group management announced on March 4th arrival of president of republic himself. Eurocopter would settle a platform welcoming several thousands of people and the president will pronounce in front of them a speech related to regional elections campaign.

One of my colleagues told me, laughing:" So you see, he brings you back your pipe…" In my deep inside, I wondered:" Why not? Anyway, that's a not-to-be-a-missed opportunity…" In this period, I already began my presidential campaign and I was seriously looking for my 500 signatures. I wanted to meet him, not as a submissive citizen, but like a challenger before a judo competition. I wanted a press photographer to freeze this moment when a handshake would unify the two rivals of the future presidential election.

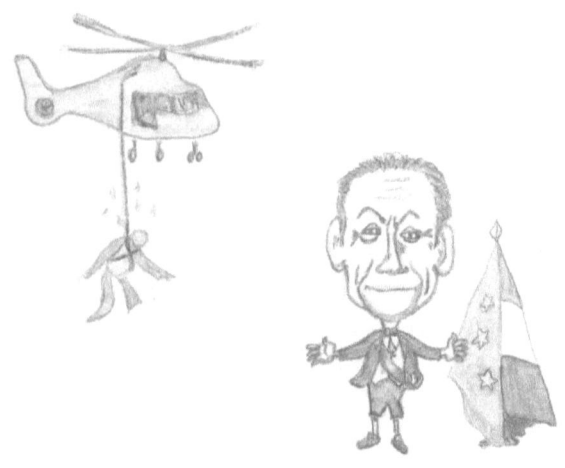

So, I sent to Eurocopter executive director an email in which I explained that first I was a candidate at the presidential election, and second I wished to shake the hand of the president during his visit. No answer from the executive director. The head of department called me and explained to me that Eurocopter site was now forbidden to me. Two days later, I was dismissed.

So, I accept for me the "ill" label. But what to say about violence of these industrial companies? Dismissed for having dared asking to shake the hand of a republic president, who is the one to be locked up?

That is the context in which, three years after his election, I grasp the president and his nasty environment who serves him blindly against me. Is it normal or not the fact I'm a bit upset against this man?

But that is not all.

In France, one often slanders African heads of state and my youth has been rocked by these sarcasms. However, there is an African country where electricity and water for domestic were free, price of a fuel per liter was 0.08€, where there were no taxes, where when a couple got married, the government provided them an apartment up to 150m2. Who could be prouder of such a social politic, of such a wealth sharing, than this African state?

On my side, I was impressed by such a social level. For sure, oil provides money to perform all these steps forward, but all the oil producers don't do it.

When I learned, a few days before my coup in Paris, that the president of republic was using French military means for exterminating this African Head of State for some dark and shameful reasons, I was terribly upset.

It's sure that my coup is a crazy action, it's sure it's very imperfectly designed, it's sure I look like Don Quichotte fighting against his mills, but what is also sure, it's that the president and all the staff around him call for people like me to be revolted.

For me, what was the stake?

My bipolar disorder was leading to heavy treatment with unpleasant side effects, especially on my sexual life. By accident, I met a Chinese medicine practitioner who proposed to me a total curation of my disease. Can I be confident in this approach? I ask my president for help, no answer. So, I try to meet with him when he comes to the site where I work. Result: I'm dismissed. And finally, he participates at the extermination of an African head of state I love very much.

In such a situation, what to do?

I try to put him away beginning an electoral campaign for presidential elections and I realize on the ground that it will be totally impossible to gather the necessary 500 signatures I need to become a true candidate.

Finally, trying to throw him away physically, was it such bad idea?

I mean, my brain tried to find a solution in the crazy world, as all ways of the real and normal world have been unsuccessfully explored.

And a lesson of such an event could be: " Unfair society should be the source of bipolar energies."

A question: this action, the coup was it finally successful?

Finally, after two months of confinement, I was back home and decided to ask for invalidity. It was accepted and this status gave me all the time to deeply think about the necessary changes in our societies. I could imagine the best way to broadcast my ideas. It also gave me time to find partners in Chinese medicine and to begin a scientific approach of this very interesting opportunity.

So, I can say: "The coup was successful".

Debriefing on a couple ending

Recently, I was in a difficult relationship with the woman I was living with. I felt that she couldn't stand any of my activities, which she was always criticizing with various excuses. She was only accepting of me from the things which were touching her directly: our walks in the country or along the seaside or our shared meals. In this context, it was difficult to imagine any kind of freedom, any kind of independency. Neither any possibility to take time to write a book, nor to work on any burning political subject, nor to be interested in any personal subject.

This state of fact made me boil. I felt I was in a cage and we were often struggling about this subject. Our domestic disputes became more and more frequent. I proposed to my girlfriend a separation. As far as I was the owner of the apartment, it was up to her to find a new roof. But, despite my insistence, she didn't want to leave.

I was trapped, submitted to unstopping criticizing, involved in a lot of disputes without any way to escape from this situation. Problem without solution. What happened?

It's very simple.

My sleep duration decreased from eight hours to less than four hours by night. Manic crisis was announced. I knew I'd have to react in order not to slide. One more time, I asked my girlfriend to go to her daughter's house for a while, time for me to manage the emotional states related to the crisis. She didn't estimate the situation's heaviness and refused one more time to leave.

For me, the situation was becoming critical. I knew the difficulty to manage the manic states of mind when alone, but there, in the climate of a disputing couple, that 'd lead me to the confinement without any doubt. So, I anticipated. I finally declared to my sticking woman: «If you don't leave, I'll confine myself to the hospital…" I was serious and she had left me with no other solution.

But this time, she understood it was serious and that there was no other solution than to leave. She did it and I thank her very much for having this smartness, for giving me this act of true love. A few days after, always floating in my manic states, I took the decision to prolongate indefinitely this separation, to put an end to this relation. The decision was not anymore smooth and hesitating, as it probably was before. No, the decision seemed to fall from the sky, urgent, imperative and mandatory.

In this very special state of mind, I informed my girlfriend about my decision to separate. This time, she understood and it's at this very precise moment that, suddenly, my sleep went back to its normal cycle of eight hours a night.

One more time, we see an example that beginning of a maniac phase brings a solution to a problem which seemed unsolvable. If I'd not turned to mania mode, maybe this domestic dispute would have lasted, and only God knows what would have happened.

How does bipolarity work?

Some people take bipolarity as a tragic disease. It's not, in my case. On the contrary, I think that bipolarity is essentially an opportunity to find solutions to unsolvable problems. I showed how it happened for three of my crises in precedent chapters.

How does it work?
Bipolarity appears when all trials for solving a problem have been unsuccessfully performed. No way to solve, but a very stressing and unpleasant problem in your life. Bipolar process extends the field of investigation. It disinhibits the person. So, it allows new ways which were forbidden before. People around are surprised because the (ill) person has a new behavior, he is not the same as usual.

To solve his problem, which has no solution in the rational world, the bipolar breaks reasonable taboo and offers to himself the luxury of madness. The problem can find a new exploration axis in this extended world of irrationality. Sometimes a solution can be found. And then, it's up to the bipolar to find a way to come back to reality with it.

Bipolar crisis breaks down the rationality scope, allows sliding and madness which open new perspectives. New ways are possible, which escape from human understanding. Coherencies still exist, but out of the usual framework. People around are afraid because the bipolar is not still in his usual behavior and tries new ways, despite caring from family and friends.

In my case, crises solved the set problems. For my couple difficulties, in two occasions, it leads to a separation. For my coup, it globally reorganized my life in a better way, with a lot of time to think about politics and to investigate Chinese medicine potential.

So, is really bipolarity a disorder?

I'd say the contrary. For sure, deep mania crisis are dangerous. For sure, depressive phases are uncomfortable and dangerous too. They must be controlled. But bipolarity is first a sign indicating that the bipolar is in a difficult situation. Bipolarity tries to cure the deepest woes, the most buried, the most stressful with an original and non-conventional method. The problem with bipolarity is its display, its symptoms are not always compatible with life in society. Does it mean that bipolarity is a disorder or that our society is very intolerant?

I am dismissed because I asked Eurocopter executive director to shake hand of the republic president when he comes to the site of the company. Who is ill? Who is to be confined? The dismissed or the man who dismisses?

Why does one put me in handcuffs, and tie my feet to a wooden bench with leather ropes before throwing me in a psychiatric hospital? Because I try to communicate with a tree? Where is freedom in France?

Bipolarity is a disease because the society has a narrow and normative vision of the person. It doesn't tolerate deviation, any excess or originality. Whatever the human cost, we must enter in the mold. That gives work to psychiatrists. They overfeed us medicines in order to make us enter in the template…

Part IV – And now?

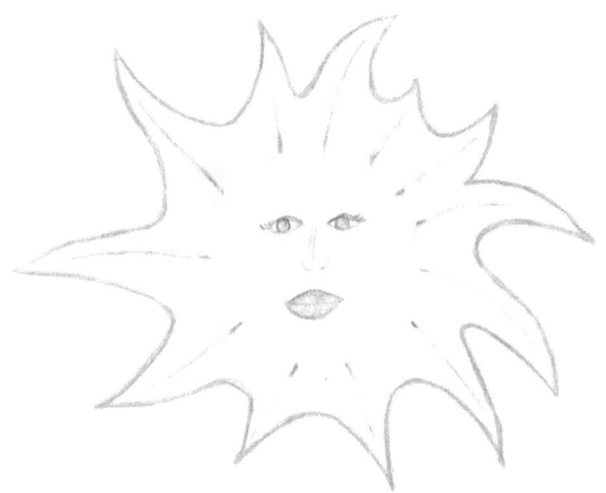

Since 1999 to 2019

In February 1999, bipolar disorder had been for us a surprise. First manic crisis had a very big impact on my life, leading to dismissal and divorce. More than ten major crises occurred since this period, which lead me to confinement every time. So, the total amount of time spent in confinement from 1999 to 2013 is about one year. In this period, treatment was not adapted or fully absent. 2013 was a turn. Treatment tuning became operational and since this date, no need of confinement.

In this period I lived many crises, many ups and downs, with all their consequences at each time, and in fact, I learned a lot. I learned about symptoms of bipolar disorder, ways to detect the crises, ways to control them. Around me, I have a team: my psychiatrist, my psychologist and different nurses ready to operate if necessary.

I have a treatment plan which lowers manic crisis occurrences. If sometimes that's not enough, I'm able to adapt the treatment in order to put out the mental fire. I'm able to recognize much earlier the beginning of a manic phase. I also know how to adapt my behavior and way of life to limit crises occurrences.

So, we can say that the situation is under control.

Moreover, I enjoy my life.

The remaining problems

"If the situation is under control and if you enjoy your life, why search further?"

There are remaining problems.

Medicines have side effects. Sexual life is not perfect, inspiration could be inhibited and renal function can be damaged. That is not nothing and reducing the treatment is a real challenge. More, I have the will to become myself again, not to be the man tuned by any medicine.

But reducing the treatment is not simple. My psychiatrist and I made several trials in the past years, reducing the Risperdal dosage from 3mg to 2mg. Each time, after a period of less than two months, I entered in a crisis.

What to do?

So, what to do?

My experience, described in detail in this book, shows that crises doesn't occur as a result of a random process, but responding to stimulating contexts. So, what to do? Simply, working on the context, on the environment, on the way of life in order to manage the contexts.

This means I've to work on my serenity, I've not to let my mind stockpile angriness seeds. I've to invent little soul safety valves to throw mental pressure when it's too high. I must know myself better. The way will be long.

I've to consider context of my first crisis: management of women desires. For that I have a roadmap. Don't submit if I'm not really in love with the person. Live the relationship with intent. But don't hesitate to break it off if it becomes a source of permanent frustrations.

Find the right way to live my politic thoughts. Try my ideas on a small group of people. Write books and listen to what people have to say.

For the bipolar disorder curation, try other techniques, try to find other partners.

And always stay prudent and don't lose what I have already acquired these last years...

The right partner

I found the right partner accidentally. Her name is Michele. Her daughter was looking for mathematics lessons and a common friend gave her my phone number. When I met her for her daughter's first lesson, she explained to me that she specialized in Chinese medicine and hypnosis. Also, in addiction management.

Immediately, I told her my problem of alcoholism. At this period, I was drinking about two bottles of wine plus two whiskies a day. I told her about my bipolarity disorder too. In fact, my psychiatrist was very anxious of my alcohol consumption because my liver was beginning to send signs of tiredness.

She answered that we could begin by treating the problem of alcohol and then pass to the bipolar disorder aspect. I said I was very interested in the proposal and asked for the price. She proposed to barter: one hour of mathematics against one hour of Chinese medicine.

I proposed to do better: we exchange the activities, but without counting anything. I'm in charge of the mathematic result of her daughter and I do my best. She's in charge of my health and she does her best. We agreed on this contract.

The alcohol

I was working on my alcoholic problem for two years with an addiction doctor, helped by shiatsu and sophrology techniques. Before Michele's intervention, we arrive to diminish sensibly my consumption but with huge mental efforts on my side. However, my consumption level is still too high. In the morning, beginning at about 10a.m., I was dreaming of my noon whisky.

Michele began by a two hours interview, followed by a session including simultaneously:
- Acupuncture
- Hypnosis
- Eye Movement Desensitization Reprocessing (EMDR)

The technique for hypnosis was the following. I'm invited to lay down on a bed. Then, Michele puts acupuncture needles in my skin. In headphones, I hear a special record which is not the same at each session. In front of my eyes, projected on special glasses, EMDR scenarios. These are colored lights moving according to the hypnosis speech.

As a result of the first session, my consumption drops from a bottle to a glass by meal and without any effort. Amazing!

Michele proposes to practice one session a week. I accept.

She also proposes a Chinese drug treatment to take for about one month. I accept.

First month, results are stable, but after this period, consumption increases again. I'm anxious.

On March 21st, a spring day, Michele proposes an interview before the session. During the hypnosis session, I decide to entirely stop alcohol. 5 months ago. Since this date, I've not drunk a drop of alcohol. And without any effort.

Day after day, the quality of my life improves. I am not thinking anymore about alcohol. I am more open, more awaken. I am not anymore hidden behind my bottle of wine, I am facing life, and I enjoy it very much.

I'm very grateful to Michele who helped me stop alcohol. I'm conscious of the power of her skills.

Bipolar disorder

So, now we are concerned by bipolar disorder curation.

Method is the same as for alcohol: acupuncture, hypnosis, EMDR and Chinese drug treatment.

In June, after six months of her treatment, we proposed to my psychiatrist a decrease of 1/3 in the Risperdal from 3mg to 2mg. She accepted giving us the advice to be extremely vigilant about crisis start.

2 months have passed, and all the indicators are good. Mind is active, but clear. Sleep has been very correct for two months. We have now a little problem certainly due to jet lag. The lack of sleep is compensated by huge moments of rest all along the day.

I notice a very good improvement of my inspiration and efficiency at writing my books. Libido is higher and sexual life is much better at 2mg than at 3mg.

So, we notice that it is the first time that we diminish Risperdal for two months and that the mind is stable, active and clear.

I think it's a good sign.

We agreed on six months platform to study each step of Risperdal decrease. So, we'll see in December if our approach is correct.

The projects

So now, what are the projects of life?

There are many.

Two projects of books. The first one is about the society without money. The aim is to show all the disadvantages due to the present exchange system and to propose a new one. The book will be a fiction. The second one will be written if our work with Michele becomes successful. In this case, we'll explain the detailed process and try to give understanding elements.

I've also projects in footpaths creation in Provence, and homeless housing too.

But the most important one is elsewhere…

I'm in love with an extraordinary woman. Her name is Deborah. I know her for two months. She lives in America and I live in Provence. I've never had such strong feelings with any woman. Our love is shared. We have a real challenge at building a life together.

Some people say it's impossible to live with a bipolar. We'll prove the contrary.

For the precise moment, please notice that she highly helped me at writing the English version of this book you're reading.

I wish to everybody to be as happy as we are...

Enjoy your life!

Thanks

Thanks to you, **Corinne**, who was my wife during critical periods. We lived together for 23 years and you had to stand my special personality. I thank you very much for your love and patience. I thank you too for having taken care of our three children, of their health and education during my illness periods. You are entirely responsible of their success and balance. I'm very grateful to you for that.

Thank you so much to you **Laura, Natacha and Guillaume**, my three children of love. My illness has been very difficult for you. Special thanks to you who had to manage my confinements against my will several times. You were very young and that was not easy at all. I'm sure that this experience, even if it has been very hard, gave you skills and understanding in human behavior. Congratulations for your success in life.

Thank you, **Mom**, for your support and understanding during all my crises. Thank you also for having given to me the day of my birth such an optimistic state of mind and ability to enjoy life.

Thank you **Maminou** and all the team from Cevennes. Your support has been very gentle and attentive. And special thanks to **Alain**, who knows how to listen to a man in manic crisis and how to give him precious advice.

Thank you, **Philippe, my GroJu**. We are friends for nearly 50 years and we always spent very intense moments together. In my illness, you always have been the rock, the one I can count on, the faithful. Thank you for that. I know that in your mind I've never been ill, but only special. This breath of fresh air is so good for me.

Thank you, **Hélène**. You are my psychiatrist for about ten years. I especially thank you because ten years ago, I was looking for a psychiatrist in order to help me at managing my mental illness. As I didn't want to take any medicine, all psychiatrists of the area refused to help me. All except you. Thank you, Hélène. You accepted me as I was, refusing the medicine. We have exchanged a lot. And finally, after months of discussion, I accepted to initiate a treatment. Thank you for being so close, for listening to me, and always trying to find solutions to my problems.

Thank you, **Bernard,** for having been a very attentive nurse during my confinements in Valvert. Thank you too for your lessons in sophrology, which have been very interesting, and are very useful in my everyday life.

Thank you to all **Valvert** psychiatric hospital staff and Aubagne Psychological Medical Center (**CMP**) staff who help me at managing my crises with great competence.

Thank you, all my companions of hospitalization. We shared difficult moments, but that was a pleasure to know you and to exchange with you. Special thanks to you, **Laurent** whose humor was so great as our time in hospital was running full speed. Congratulations for your very impressive caritative actions. I'm very proud to have you as a friend.

Thank you, **Etienne, Lucile and Delphine**, and to all the team of the Addictology center (**CSAPA**) of Aubagne. Your help in my struggle against alcohol was essential.

Thank you **Michèle.** Chinese medicine and hypnosis practitioner, you are responsible for a huge improvement in my life. Because of your help and skills, I stopped drinking alcohol. Now, we are already able to reduce Risperdal treatment by 1/3. This improves greatly my quality of life. I thank you so much and I wish you very great professional success.

Thank you, **Stacie** for having been present 20 years ago through very difficult moments of my life. Thank you for your care and attention. Thank you too for helping me with this book improvement by a meticulous review. Thank you for being a very precious friend.

Thank you, **Deborah**, my great love. Your participation in this book was huge. Exchanging with me very frequently, you helped me a lot at structuring my thoughts and ideas. Your influence led to a complete reorganization of the plan for more readability and clearness. In our everyday life, you have a great flexibility and you accommodate easily with specialties of my illness. For that, you are an exception. My life with you is a wonderful dream. I've never lived such a happiness. Thank you for all that, Deborah…

Table of contents

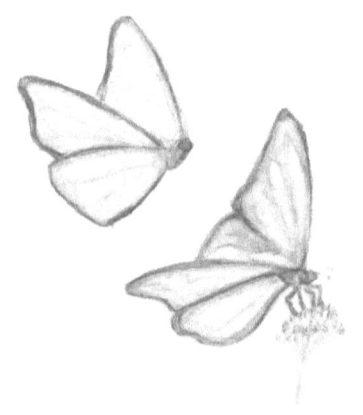

Dépôt légal : septembre 2019